PSOAS
Strength and Flexibility

PSOAS
Strength and Flexibility

Core Workouts to Increase Mobility, Reduce Injuries and End Back Pain

Pamela Ellgen, CPT

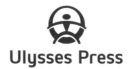

Ulysses Press

Published in the United States by
Ulysses Press
P.O. Box 3440
Berkeley, CA 94703
www.ulyssespress.com

ISBN: 978-1-61243-432-2

Library of Congress Control Number 2014952016

Printed in the United States by Bang Printing

10 9 8 7 6 5 4 3 2 1

Acquisitions: Keith Riegert
Managing editor: Claire Chun
Editor: Lily Chou
Proofreader: Renee Rutledge
Indexer: Sayre Van Young
Front cover/interior design and layout: what!design @ whatweb.com
Artwork: cover © leonello calvetti/shutterstock.com; page 6 © stihii/shutterstock.com
Models: Nadia Brunner-Velasquez, Pamela Ellgen, Bryan Johnson

Distributed by Publishers Group West

Please Note: This book has been written and published strictly for informational purposes, and in no way should be used as a substitute for consultation with health care professionals. You should not consider educational material herein to be the practice of medicine or to replace consultation with a physician or other medical practitioner. The author and publisher are providing you with information in this work so that you can have the knowledge and can choose, at your own risk, to act on that knowledge. The author and publisher also urge all readers to be aware of their health status and to consult health care professionals before beginning any health program.

This book is independently authored and published. No sponsorship or endorsement of this book by, and no affiliation with any trademarked brands or products mentioned or pictured, is claimed or suggested. All trademarks that appear in this book belong to their respective owners and are used here for informational purposes only. The author and publisher encourage readers to patronize the quality brands and other products mentioned and pictured in this book.

To my sons, Brad and Cole

Table of Contents

Part 1: OVERVIEW 1

Introduction 2

What Is the Psoas? 4

Is Your Psoas Healthy? 8

Maintaining a Healthy Psoas 12

Nutrition & Weight Loss 19

Part 2: FLEXIBILITY EXERCISES   27

Active Stretches 28

Leg Swing 29   Lunge 33
Walking Psoas Stretch 30   Inner Thigh Stretch 34
Kneeling Knee Crunch 32

Static Stretches 35

Static Kneeling Psoas Stretch 36   Quadriceps Stretch 42
Bent-Knee Stretch.............................38   Hamstrings Stretch 43
Hamstrings Stretch on Bench 39   Kneeling Psoas Stretch with Leg Rotation...........44
Bent-Knee Stretch on Roller 40   Kneeling Wall Stretch 46
Outer Thigh Stretch 41

Self-Myofascial Release 47

Psoas Release....................................49   Hamstrings Release 52
Piriformis & Gluteal Muscles Release.......50   Quadriceps Release 53
Outer Front Hip Release 51

Yoga 54

Corpse Pose 56   Bridge Pose 62
Mountain Pose 57   Triangle Pose 63
Tree Pose 58   Cobra Pose 64
Pigeon Pose 60   Crow Pose 65
Boat Pose 61   Standing Big Toe Pose 66

Pilates 68

Pelvic Curl 71   Roll-Up 76
Supine Leg Lift 72   Neck Pull 77
Prone Back Extension.......................73   Hundred 78
One-Leg Circle 74   Single Bent-Leg Stretch 79

Single Straight-Leg Stretch 80
Double-Leg Stretch 81
Teaser...................................... 82
Open-Leg Rocker 83
Rollover 84

Jackknife 86
Scissors 87
Spine Twist 88
Corkscrew 90

Part 3: STRENGTH EXERCISES   91

Strength Training.............................92

Chair V-Sit 93
Scissors 94
Captain's Chair 95
Plank....................................... 96
Opposite Arm & Leg Raise 97
Russian Twist 98
Cat-Cow Pose 99
Superman 100
Extension on Exercise Ball 101
Side Plank................................. 102

Dead Lift 104
Standing Side Kick......................... 106
Single-Leg Hip Lift 108
Knee Extension 109
Single-Leg Squat with Reverse Wood Chop 110
Static Wall Squat 112
Side-Lying Clamshell 114
Quadruped Leg Lift with Bent Leg 115
Quadruped Leg Lift with Straight Leg 116

Part 4: PROGRAMS   117

Psoas Programs 118

General Psoas Flexibility 119
General Psoas Strength 120

Psoas Strength & Flexibility
for Sedentary Population 121

Psoas Healing from Pain,
Swelling & Spasms........................... 122

References 123

Index 129

Acknowledgments 133

About the Author 135

Part 1: OVERVIEW

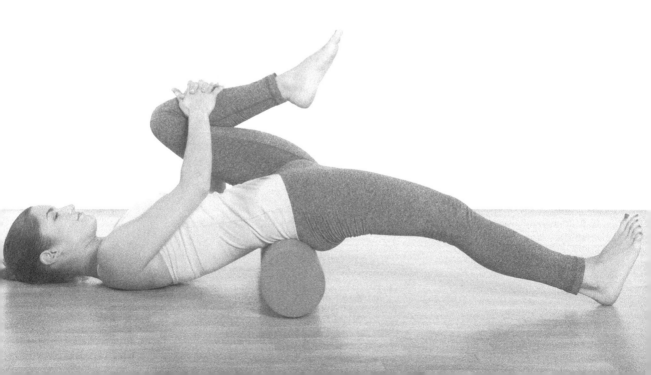

Introduction

Walk into any gym in America and you'll find endless rows of equipment to train your arms, back, core, and legs. But where's the machine for strengthening your psoas? The showpiece muscles get all the attention while the psoas goes unnoticed.

Fitness magazines are equally dismissive. It's amusing to even imagine the headlines they might come up with: "10 Tips for Shaping Up Your Psoas" or "Get a Beach-Ready Psoas by Summer!"

However, the psoas' lack of exposure is no indication of its importance in your physical health and fitness. In fact, the effects of a tight or weak psoas can be substantial, including poor posture, a protruding stomach, hip and knee pain, and decreased mobility.

This book aims to help you develop a healthy psoas muscle. First, it will help you evaluate the health of your psoas and determine whether it's shortened and tight or lengthened and weak; however, none of these conditions is mutually exclusive. All can be affected by various lifestyle factors, including weight, body-fat composition, non-exercise activity level, fitness, nutrition, sleep, and hydration.

Part 1 discusses the ways in which these factors contribute to psoas health or dysfunction as well as complementary medical treatments for psoas health. It also provides nutrition and lifestyle recommendations to facilitate healthy hip flexors.

Part 2 focuses on flexibility exercises, including yoga and Pilates, that improve range of motion in your hip flexors, abdominal muscles, and lower back. It also features tension-soothing self-myofascial release techniques that target fascial adhesions.

Part 3 is dedicated to providing resistance exercises to build strength in the quadriceps, gluteal muscles, hamstrings, abdominal muscles, and lumbar spine, all of which contribute to the healthy functioning of your psoas muscle so it works synergistically with the surrounding muscles.

Part 4 provides focused programs for specific concerns, including workouts for people who are sedentary or seeking relief from pain and swelling.

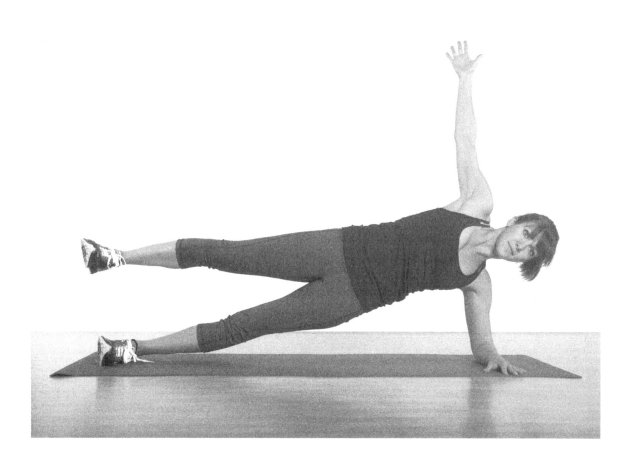

What Is the Psoas?

The psoas major is a muscle that wraps around your pelvis from your lower back forward to the lower part of your pelvis at the inner thigh of both legs. More specifically, it originates at the anterior lateral aspect of the lumbar vertebrae L5, joins the iliacus in the pelvis, and inserts at the lesser trochanter of the femur. Imagine a bikini bottom from the 1980s with its high leg cut and you have a general idea of where the psoas muscle lies, though it does not join at the pubis but attaches to the femur. Together, the psoas and iliacus muscles are referred to as the iliopsoas.

The psoas major is long and wide at its midline, with a conical shape on each end; it's what is known as a fusiform muscle. It's composed of slow- and fast-twitch muscle fibers, meaning it's capable of both sustaining endurance activities at low levels of intensity and producing bursts of movement for a short duration. In about 50 percent of humans, the psoas major is also joined by a very thin muscle called the psoas minor.

The iliopsoas is part of a larger muscle group called the hip flexors. These include the rectus femoris and sartorius located on the front of your thigh, the tensor fasciae latae, which is part of your hip and upper thigh muscles, and the pectineus, adductor longus, adductor brevis, and gracilis, which are all part of your medial thigh.

Function of the Psoas

Although you can't see your psoas muscle, it's literally at the center of most of your everyday movement, from walking or bending over to twisting and reaching. In conjunction with the other hip flexors, the psoas is responsible for bringing the upper thigh toward the torso or bringing the torso toward the thigh, depending on whether your legs or spine is stationary. The psoas also participates in the rotation of the trunk and external rotation of the hip joint.

Here are some of the daily movements and exercises that involve the psoas:

o Walking

o Climbing stairs

o Running

o Cycling

o Sit-ups and crunches

No skeletal muscle in your body functions independently. All work synergistically to produce movement, maintain posture, and stabilize joints. Muscles that cause movement by contracting are called agonists. A muscle is considered an antagonist when it resists a particular movement. A synergist muscle is one that helps an agonist or antagonist accomplish movement or stabilization. Synergist muscles also help control movement, holding a particular joint in place so that an action can be accomplished without injury.

For the iliopsoas, muscle synergists include the pectineus, tensor fasciae latae, adductor brevis, and sartorius. Additional synergists include the adductor longus and anterior portion of the adductor magnus, gracilis, gluteus minimus, and quadratus lumborum. Antagonists include the gluteus maximus and the posterior portion of the adductor magnus.

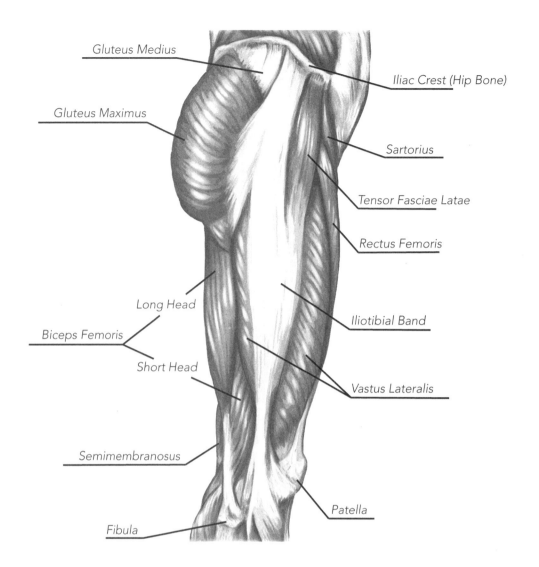

Gluteus Medius

Iliac Crest (Hip Bone)

Gluteus Maximus

Sartorius

Tensor Fasciae Latae

Rectus Femoris

Long Head

Iliotibial Band

Biceps Femoris

Short Head

Vastus Lateralis

Semimembranosus

Patella

Fibula

All of these muscles are involved, to varying degrees, in the healthy functioning of the iliopsoas in all planes of motion. Thus, all must be strong, flexible, and balanced (none displaying dominance) for the psoas muscle to perform optimally. If one is out of alignment or weak, it will necessarily compromise the functioning of another portion of the kinetic chain.

KINETIC CHAIN: *A combination of several successively arranged joints constituting a complex motor unit in which the movement of each joint affects the movement of another joint within the kinetic link.*

Is the Psoas Really that Important?

While the psoas muscle is active in most of your everyday movement and stationary behavior, it's possible to overstate its importance. In fact, some authors have. Liz Koch, self-proclaimed psoas aficionado and author of *The Psoas Book*, says, "The only muscle to connect your spine to your leg, the psoas influences everything from low back pain and anxiety to full-body orgasms and pure pleasure." She goes on to say, "A tense psoas can disturb digestion, reproductive functioning and create a host of other aliments [sic]. Released and vital it fosters feelings of pleasure and comfortable [sic]."

Although that approach might sell books, it oversimplifies the myriad factors that affect human physiology and overlooks the function of the psoas within the context of the kinetic chain.

That's not what this book is about. However, though the psoas isn't the key to unlocking the mysteries of sexual satisfaction or mental illness, a tight or weak psoas does have a profound effect on functional movement and can contribute to pain, postural problems, and muscle imbalances. When flexible and strong, it facilitates healthy functioning in daily movement, recreation, and exercise. All strength and flexibility exercises contained herein seek to train the psoas within the context of the kinetic chain for a holistic approach to the health of your hip flexors, abdominal muscles, and lumbar spine.

Is Your Psoas Healthy?

Various lifestyle factors impact your hip mobility and the health of your psoas. Sitting for long periods of time—a reality for many people in office settings—can contribute to a tight psoas muscle. Various sports can also contribute to irritation and inflammation of the psoas and lead to a condition known as iliopsoas syndrome, which affects both the tendon attaching the psoas to the hip bone and the iliopsoas bursa, a fluid-filled sac that provides a cushion between the tendon and hip joint. Runners, dancers, and gymnasts are at particular risk due to extensive hip flexion. Additionally, constant sit-ups and cycling can contribute to psoas overuse injuries.

Developing a healthy psoas muscle requires more than simply stretching it or strengthening it. Think of your skeletal muscles as guitar strings. Before you begin to play, you make sure the instrument is in tune and then adjust it accordingly. If you were to simply tighten all of the strings, it wouldn't be more in tune; some strings would be more in tune but others would be less. The same goes for loosening all of the strings. You first have to determine whether each string is playing slightly sharp or flat and then adjust accordingly. The same can be said of your skeletal muscles. They may be tight and require stretching, or weak and require strengthening, or a combination of both.

So, how do you know what your psoas needs? There are a few ways to test for psoas health.

Evaluating Psoas Flexibility: Modified Thomas Test

The Thomas Test involves lying on your back on an examination table or a mat on the floor and bringing one knee in toward your chest until your lower back flattens and your knee grazes your abdomen. The remaining leg remains extended. If the straight leg elevates just below the hip, you likely have a tight psoas muscle. If the straight leg bends at the knee, you likely have a tight rectus femoris, which is part of your quadriceps.

STARTING POSITION: Lie on the floor with your spine straight and your legs extended hip-width apart. Relax your back, neither arching it nor pressing your lower back into the floor. Allow it to curve naturally.

1: Using your hands to guide and assist, slowly bring one knee in toward your chest until you feel your lower back flatten.

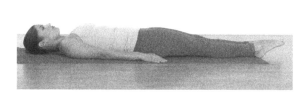 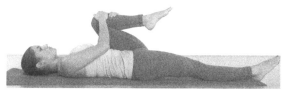

Observe your extended leg carefully. The move will cause your pelvis to tilt slightly, but if the psoas muscle is optimally lengthened, it won't elevate the upper thigh or force your knee to bend. If either of these occur, flexibility should be part of your psoas training program.

Evaluating Psoas Strength: Standing Wall Test

Your psoas is partially responsible for flexing your hips. However, a tight psoas is not the same thing as a strong psoas. Testing for psoas strength involves flexing your hip for an extended period of time to see whether the psoas tires quickly. Make sure you're wearing loose clothing; tight pants will confound the results and suggest weakness or inflexibility where it may not exist.

STARTING POSITION: Stand with your back against a wall and your feet hip-width apart.

1: Slowly elevate one knee toward your chest until your upper thigh is parallel with the floor. Hold the position for 30 seconds.

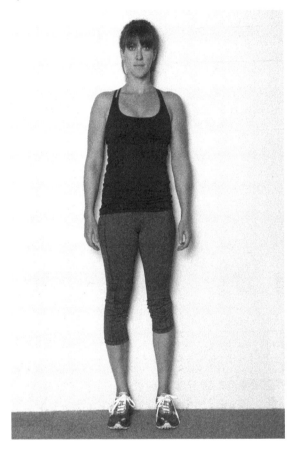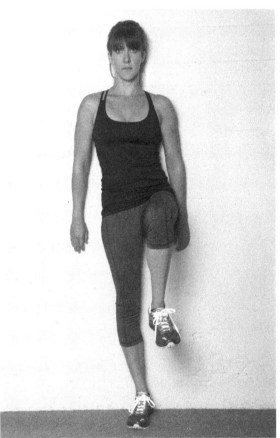

If you're able to do this easily, your psoas and its synergist muscles are likely strong.

Psoas Syndrome

Psoas syndrome, characterized by lower back pain, difficulty maintaining proper posture, and pain radiating down one leg, is an easily missed diagnosis, according to an article published in *The Journal of the American Osteopathic Association*. Some of the difficulty in diagnosing psoas syndrome stems from the fact that many other conditions, some of them quite serious, could be responsible for the symptoms. If you suspect that you have psoas syndrome, don't attempt to treat it on your own. Instead, seek proper medical evaluation and treatment. Part of that treatment may involve at-home stretching and strengthening exercises, but these should be overseen by your physician. Left untreated, psoas syndrome can contribute to restriction of the diaphragm and even disability beyond that of other chronic back conditions, in addition to the existing symptoms.

Maintaining a Healthy Psoas

Numerous factors affect the health of your psoas muscle, but your daily movement, or lack thereof, is the most manifest. More than the exercises you perform, the movement patterns you have throughout the day have a profound effect on the muscle.

Ergonomics

Modern life is somewhat inconducive to a healthy psoas muscle. Most of our lives are built around one posture—sitting. We drive to work, sit down at work, drive home, sit down to eat, and then sit down to put our feet up for a little television. All of that sitting leaves our psoas in a shortened position for hours on end.

The psoas isn't the only casualty of extended periods of sitting. The habit has far-reaching effects, increasing your risks for becoming overweight or obese, type 2 diabetes, cardiovascular disease, cancer, and early death.

If you work in an office setting, there are several steps you can take to change the ergonomics of your workstation to improve your psoas health. Bonus, you may find that the changes improve workflow and productivity and help you maintain a healthy weight.

- **Consider a standing desk.** This will allow you to stand for portions of the day while maintaining productivity. You should have a counter-height chair available to sit as needed since standing all day can lead to pain in your lower back, knees, and feet.

- **Skip sending e-mail to colleagues** within the office and get up to go visit them. A study published in the journal *Science* found that those who spent more of their day fidgeting, standing, or walking burned 350 more calories throughout the day than those who remained sedentary. Both groups were fed 1,000 more calories and told not to engage in formal exercise. Only the fidgety group successfully avoided weight gain. This and other studies have confirmed that movement throughout the day is more valuable than single bouts of exercise on top of an otherwise sedentary lifestyle.

- **Don't trade your office chair for an exercise or stability ball.** Despite what fitness commercials and well-meaning gym-goers may tell you, sitting on a fitness ball for office work not only doesn't burn many additional calories or activate your abdominal muscles, it may actually decrease psoas length and require constant contraction to maintain the posture.

- **Perform several psoas stretches throughout the day** if sitting all day is unavoidable. Some of the best choices include Standing and Walking Lunges (page 33), Quadriceps Stretch (page 42), Tree Pose (page 58), and Chair V-Sit (page 93).

These require no special equipment or extensive space, nor do they require you to lie on the floor, which may be undesirable in an office setting.

If you do have an office job or an otherwise sedentary occupation, make sure to evaluate your psoas health using the strength and flexibility tests described on page 9.

Exercise

Simply staying active will improve the health of your psoas muscle due to increased blood circulation, improved oxygen delivery, and greater joint and muscle mobility. In addition to the prescriptive exercises suggested in this book, incorporate more movement into your everyday life, especially if you have a sedentary occupation. Aim for 30–60 minutes daily of moderate-intensity cardiovascular exercise on most if not all days of the week, along with 20–30 minutes of strength training three days per week.

Exercise need not involve endless sessions on the treadmill. There are so many pleasurable ways to increase your physical activity level. Consider adding one or two of these recreational activities to your existing routine:

Archery	Golf	Stand-up paddleboarding
Basketball	Handball	Surfing
Bowling	Hiking	Swimming
Canoeing	Horseback riding	Tennis
Croquet	Martial arts	Volleyball
Cycling	Rock climbing	Water aerobics
Dancing	Rowing	Zumba
Fencing	Skiing or Snowboarding	
Frisbee	Soccer	

Both for recreation and deliberate physical fitness training, choose a variety of activities. Not only does this help stave off boredom, it also develops greater range of motion and prevents sport-specific muscle imbalances and overuse injuries. Ultimately, whatever exercise you find enjoyable and are most likely to engage in is the best exercise to use for aerobic activity.

STRENGTH TRAINING

According to the American Council on Exercise, a regular strength-training routine has numerous positive effects:

o Increased strength of bones, muscles, and connective tissues

o Decreased risk of injury

o Increased muscle mass and basal metabolic rate

o Enhanced quality of life

Strength training should include resistance exercise for all major muscle groups and be done with proper form to reduce the risk of muscle imbalances and injury. Multi-joint functional movements such as squats and push-ups incorporate more than one muscle group and develop functional strength. A personal trainer can help you create a program that challenges your whole body and addresses your particular physical and medical history.

Sleep

The importance of healthy sleep patterns cannot be overstated. Logging at least eight hours of shut-eye a night may seem like a luxury, but it's essential to your health. Adequate sleep improves hormone regulation and weight maintenance, while insufficient sleep is implicated in driving hunger and reducing satiety mechanisms as well as decreasing motivation and ability to engage in exercise. This is an unfortunate reality because exercise improves sleep quality. Lost sleep yields less exercise, which in turn yields less sleep.

Inadequate sleep may also contribute to chronic pain and decrease pain tolerance, both of which can further contribute to sleep loss. Clearly, sleep is a reciprocal issue and developing healthy sleep patterns will influence numerous positive outcomes. Here are several simple steps you can take toward developing healthy sleep habits.

ENSURE YOUR BEDROOM IS CONDUCIVE TO SLEEP. The temperature of your room should be cool, between 65–72 degrees, for optimal sleep. The room should be dark but not pitch black. Room darkening shades can help with this in addition to removing electronic devices that emit light, such as alarm clocks, phones, and even phone chargers. Air circulation from a fan may improve respiration and provide white noise to block out distractions that affect sleep quality.

ELIMINATE EVENING SCREEN TIME BEFORE BED. The blue light emitted by televisions, computers, tablets, and cell phones decreases melatonin secretion, which helps you feel sleepy. Turn off your electronic devices and LED lighting and replace them with dim, warm lighting. Even lighting candles instead of turning on an LED lamp can improve sleep quality. Just make sure to blow them out before you hit the hay.

ESTABLISH A SLEEP SCHEDULE. Sleeping and waking at the same time every day—yes, even on the weekends—will contribute to better, deeper sleep. And, when you're well rested, you won't even miss sleeping in on your day off.

GO EASY ON THE ALCOHOL. If you use a few drinks to help you fall asleep in the evening, it could be backfiring. However, a single drink may have no effect or even improve sleep quality and duration, according to research published in the journal *Electroencephalography and Clinical Neurophysiology*.

ADOPT A HEALTHY SLEEP POSTURE. Sleeping in an exaggerated fetal position contributes to psoas tightness whereas stomach sleeping may contribute to psoas lengthening and spinal lordosis. Sleep on your back or side with your spine in a neutral position.

EXERCISE EVERY DAY. Even if you don't feel like it, a small bout of exercise every day can improve sleep quality. If you're already sleep deprived and have difficulty falling asleep and staying asleep, adding exercise to your daily routine can improve sleep quality and increase your desire to engage in exercise on subsequent days.

Hydration & Your Psoas

Dehydration contributes to numerous health consequences, but its effect on skeletal muscles is rarely discussed outside of medical journals. Inadequate fluid intake is known to decrease muscular power, strength, and endurance. Its effect on posture is more subtle but equally important. A study published in the journal *Neuroscience* evaluated the effects of hydration on postural control and found that poor hydration, particularly in the presence of intense exercise, yielded poor postural regulation.

Thirst may or may not be a reliable indicator of hydration levels. Thus, developing regular hydration habits will ensure adequate fluid intake. Aim for 64–96 ounces of water daily depending on your activity level and the environment in which you live. People living at high altitudes or in arid climates, or those who engage in strenuous activity, will need greater levels of fluid.

Chiropractic Care & Massage

According to the Mayo Clinic, the goal of chiropractic adjustment is to correct structural alignment and improve functional movement. Massage therapy is considered a form of complementary medicine. Varieties of massage therapy include Swedish massage, deep tissue, sports massage, and trigger point, which vary in purpose, intensity, and the types of strokes used by the massage therapist.

Both chiropractic and massage therapy are often sought as a treatment for lower back pain and research suggests that both can be as effective as conventional treatments. Nevertheless, neither chiropractic nor massage therapy are particularly successful at manipulating the psoas muscle itself. The muscle is buried deep beneath other muscle tissue, fat, and organs. Thus, working the psoas in isolation is difficult, even for a competent massage therapist or chiropractor.

If it can be located successfully, another major challenge is that psoas work can be incredibly uncomfortable, according to former Registered Massage Therapist Paul Ingraham. "Like most flexors, the iliopsoas is quite sensitive to pressure, and the quality of pain is almost always unpleasant," he says. "It takes time and caution to do it well and without causing significant discomfort — even extreme discomfort."

Ingraham also warns against seeking treatment from practitioners who mistakenly believe that the psoas is the key to diagnosing and treating all pain and injury. "This is a classic example of 'structuralism': the excessive focus on specific biomechanical origins of pain," he says.

A better approach to massage and chiropractic care for psoas health is to use it to facilitate healthy bone, joint, and muscle functioning for all of the muscles from the lower back through the hips, butt, and thighs.

If you pursue chiropractic care, seek a recommendation from your primary care doctor or spine specialist. According to a review published in the journal *Evidence Report Technology Assessment*, some studies have found spinal manipulation is significantly associated with vertebral artery dissection, which can cause temporary or permanent stroke-like symptoms, and vertebrobasilar vascular accident. However, typically, these only occur with neck manipulation and are very rare.

Physical Therapy

A qualified physical therapist can provide effective treatment for those with psoas syndrome or symptoms of pain, swelling, spasms, or a tight or weak psoas muscle. It's especially important for people who are experiencing these symptoms to have a medical professional, such as a physical therapist, oversee their treatment and rehabilitation. A physical therapist might prescribe specific strength and flexibility exercises, external manipulation, ice, rest, medication, or a combination of these designed to address your specific condition.

Alternative Treatments

Various alternative treatments may contribute to psoas health. Some of these include acupuncture, qigong, and Structural Integration. Always check with your primary care physician before engaging in alternative treatments, especially if you're experiencing pain or discomfort, and seek a qualified practitioner.

Nutrition & Weight Loss

In addition to your daily movement patterns, what you eat and your weight affect the health of your psoas. This section contains information on how to reduce inflammation as well as achieve and maintain a healthy weight for a healthy psoas.

Inflammation

Not only is the psoas subject to damage from overuse, poor ergonomics, and other physical considerations, it's also susceptible to inflammation from stress, diet, and other lifestyle factors. Acute inflammation is a good thing—your body is rushing to the site of pain or injury to repair the damage. However, chronic inflammation is when your body is in constant "crisis intervention" mode. Some of the foods that contribute to chronic inflammation include:

WHEAT AND SUGAR. Simple carbohydrates are the worst offenders for contributing to inflammation. From bread, breakfast cereal, and pasta to sweetened drinks, pastries, and desserts, all contribute to elevated blood sugar and insulin levels, which play a role in creating a state of chronic inflammation—your body's constant "crisis intervention" mode. Even whole-wheat bread has a surprisingly high glycemic index and is implicated in contributing to inflammation. Gluten-free goods are not off the hook, either, when they replace wheat with other refined grains and sugar.

PROCESSED FOODS. Fried and overly processed foods have inflammatory effects. French fries in particular have both a high glycemic index along with fats that have oxidized due to repeated cooking at high temperatures. Processed meats such as pepperoni, lunch meat, and hot dogs are equally damaging.

OVERCOOKED MEAT. Advanced glycation end products, or AGEs, damage proteins in the body and elevate cytokines, which are inflammatory compounds. AGEs are formed in alarming quantities in meat that has been cooked for long periods of time or at high temperatures—think a well-done steak prepared on the grill.

COOKING OIL. Another dietary contributor to inflammation is industrial seed and vegetable oils—corn, canola, soybean, sunflower, and safflower oils, among others—with an unhealthy balance of omega-6 to omega-3 fatty acids.

It's not all bad news, though—many delicious foods actually help calm inflammation and reverse and repair cellular damage. Fill your grocery sack with these items to not only quell inflammation but also aid in weight loss.

VEGETABLES. Broccoli, kale, garlic, onions, spinach, bok choy, and red cabbage, among numerous others, have all shown potency in clinical trials at reducing inflammation.

BERRIES. Numerous varieties of berries have demonstrated anti-inflammatory effects in scientific studies. Choose organic or wild berries in season whenever possible. Some excellent options include blueberries, raspberries, blackberries, cranberries, goji berries, and strawberries. They are all high in fiber, antioxidants, vitamins, and minerals.

FISH. Choose salmon and other wild, sustainably harvested cold-water fish, such as European anchovies, Pacific sardines, bluefin tuna, Atlantic herring, rainbow trout, and Atlantic mackerel. If you're not a fan of fish, opt for high-quality fish oil supplements. A study published in the journal *Pharmaceutical Biology* in 2012 found that six months of fish oil supplementation improved fat metabolism and ameliorated inflammation in patients with metabolic syndrome.

NUTS AND SEEDS. Among plants, nuts (particularly walnuts, pecans, chestnuts, and peanuts) and seeds contain some of the highest concentrations of antioxidants. In 2006, the *American Journal of Epidemiology* published an analysis of data on over 6,000 US adults. Researchers observed that frequent nut and seed consumption (as many as five servings per week) was associated with lower levels of the inflammatory markers C-reactive protein, interleukin-6, and fibrinogen.

COCONUT OIL. This tropical oil derived from coconut meat is rich in antioxidants and appears to have strong anti-inflammatory effects, according to a study published in the journal *International Immunopharmacology* in 2014. Don't worry too much about coconut oil's saturated fat content. First, emerging research and a reanalysis of the research that first led us to fear it in the first place suggests that it may not be as bad for our health as previously thought. Moreover, 50 percent of the saturated fat in coconut oil is lauric acid, which has antiviral and antibacterial properties.

SPICES. Turmeric, ginger, and red pepper all have potent anti-inflammatory effects. Turmeric and ginger both reduced the incidence and severity of arthritis in a clinical trial conducted in 2011 and published in the journal *Inflammation*. Fortunately, a little goes a long way, so consider adding a teaspoon of turmeric or ginger to your morning smoothie or evening stirfry.

Body Composition

Developing the strength and flexibility of your psoas provides yet another reason to achieve and maintain a healthy weight and body-fat composition. When overweight or obesity occurs in an individual, excess fat exists not only in protruding stomachs and thighs but also in and around your skeletal muscles. This is what scientists call intramuscular adipose tissue, or IMAT. Even if your body mass index is within a healthy range (18.5–25), an elevated ratio of body fat to lean muscle tissue will contribute to increased IMAT deposits.

The consequences of IMAT include insulin resistance, loss of strength, and impaired mobility.

A review published in the *International Journal of Endocrinology* in 2011 found that IMAT is a significant predictor of muscle strength and mobility. The review included a cross section of the thighs of two female subjects with the same body mass index and muscle size. One woman displayed twice the IMAT, 18.8 cm compared to 9.8 cm, than the other woman. The woman with the greater IMAT showed a 45 percent decrease in leg power and a 24 percent decrease in leg strength, suggesting that intramuscular fat deposits have severe consequences on physical function even with the same volume of muscle.

Body-Fat Percentage		
	Women	Men
Essential fat	10–13%	2–5%
Athletes	14–20%	6–13%
Fitness	21–24%	14–17%
Average	25–31%	18–24%
Obese	32% +	25% +

Source: American Council on Exercise

Fortunately, reductions in overall weight typically result in commensurate reductions in IMAT. A study published in 2014 in the journal *Clinical Interventions in Aging* found that an 8 percent decrease in body weight after a combined diet and exercise intervention yielded a 9 percent decrease in IMAT around the psoas muscle.

Weight Loss

Both diet and exercise contribute to weight loss and both are necessary for successful, sustained weight loss. However, what you eat often plays a greater role than your workout—particularly in the short term.

The most effective nutrition strategies for weight loss focus on whole foods and include an abundance of unprocessed, sustainably harvested plant and animal foods—the types of food that humans have thrived on for millennia. According to an article published in *The American Journal of Clinical Nutrition*, the Neolithic and Industrial periods (beginning at about 10,000 B.C. and the middle of the 18th century, respectively) introduced foods and processing methods that altered several critical elements present in the human diet up until that time: the glycemic load, fatty acid composition, macronutrient content (protein, fat, and carbohydrates), micronutrient density, sodium-potassium ratio, and fiber content. These changes resulted in numerous consequences for human health, notably overweight and obesity.

Although primitive diets varied widely by geographic region, season, and availability, they all had this in common: minimally processed wild plant and animal foods. Numerous popular weight-loss programs offer interpretations of ancestral approaches to food, nutrition, and weight loss, including the Paleo Diet, the Primal Blueprint, and Whole30. Each has its own unique style and strategies, but all eliminate inflammatory foods and allow your body to shed excess pounds without counting calories or excessive feelings of hunger. All of these approaches are decidedly low-carb, which research confirms is more effective than low-fat diets for long-term weight loss.

What to Avoid

An ancestral eating plan eliminates grains and legumes, dairy, refined sugar, and industrial oils. For many Americans, this comprises their entire menu: cereal with low-fat milk and orange juice for breakfast, light popcorn for a snack, a peanut butter sandwich on whole wheat with a diet Coke for lunch, and a frozen packaged meal for dinner with a slice of low-fat chocolate cake for dessert. It has earned the unfortunate moniker SAD, Standard American Diet, for the devastating effects it has had on our waistlines and our health. Restricting calories within the SAD paradigm may yield some weight loss, but it typically results in nagging hunger, constant cravings, fatigue, irritability, and failure to lose a significant amount of weight. If the vast number of diets on the market and our escalating problem with overweight and obesity is any indication, dieting within this paradigm simply doesn't work.

What to Eat

Modern interpretations of the ancestral eating pattern include plenty of fresh, seasonal vegetables, sustainably raised and harvested meat, fish, poultry, and pastured eggs, along with some fresh fruit, nuts and seeds, and healthy fats from coconut and olive oils. Herbs, spices, coffee, dark chocolate, and wine are also included in some contemporary versions of an ancestral diet. Counting calories is unnecessary when you're eating this way because your body's built-in mechanisms become reliable indicators of hunger and satiety. Processed foods, grains, and dairy easily override these signals. Nevertheless, the rise in popularity of ancestral diets has given way to many foods (baked goods and desserts in particular) that are technically within the framework of ancestral foods but are inconducive to weight loss.

FRESH VEGETABLES. Enjoy 5–10 servings a day of fresh, seasonal vegetables. Purchase organic whenever possible and prudent—if the organic produce is wilting on store shelves, conventional may be a better option. Choose mostly non-starchy vegetables.

Artichoke	Celery	Lettuce
Arugula	Chard	Mushroom
Asparagus	Collard greens	Onion
Beets	Cucumber	Pepper
Bok choy	Garlic	Radish
Broccoli	Green beans	Squash
Brussels sprouts	Herbs	Sweet potato
Carrots	Kale	Tomato
Cauliflower	Leek	Watercress

FRESH FRUITS. Enjoy up to 2 servings of fruit daily when you're trying to lose weight, or up to 4 servings daily for weight maintenance. Berries are one of the most nutritious options with the least amount of sugar.

Apple	Currant	Orange
Apricot	Fig	Peach
Avocado	Grape	Pear
Banana	Grapefruit	Plum/prune
Blackberry	Kiwi fruit	Pineapple
Blueberry	Lemon	Pomegranate
Boysenberry	Lime	Raspberry
Breadfruit	Marionberry	Strawberry
Cantaloupe	Melon	Watermelon
Cherry	Nectarine	

MEAT AND POULTRY. Choose organic, grass-fed, or pastured meat and poultry whenever possible. They're typically leaner and contain more nutrients than conventionally raised animals.

Beef	Lamb	Pork
Chicken	Organ meats	Turkey

FISH AND SEAFOOD. Choose sustainably caught wild seafood for most of your purchases. The Monterey Bay Aquarium's Seafood Watch offers recommendations for the best choices for sustainable seafood.

Clam	Halibut	Salmon
Cod	Mussel	Shrimp

OTHER PROTEIN SOURCES. Eggs, nuts, and seeds provide additional options for muscle-building amino acids. Choose pastured eggs whenever possible and choose raw nuts over those that have been roasted in polyunsaturated fatty acids, which can contribute to inflammation.

Almond	Sesame seed	Whole egg
Hazelnut	Walnut	

Supplements

Most of the nutrients your body needs to stay healthy and feel energized should come from whole foods. However, sometimes supplementation can be helpful to correct existing nutrient deficiencies or if you're consuming overly processed or non-organic, conventionally farmed foods, which have lower nutritional value than organic, sustainably raised, or wild harvested foods.

OMEGA-3 FATTY ACID. Supplementing with omega-3 fats may reduce inflammation and symptoms of joint pain, particularly when it's associated with rheumatoid arthritis and osteoporosis.

MAGNESIUM AND POTASSIUM. The mineral magnesium plays a critical role in muscle relaxation, and magnesium deficiency can contribute to potassium deficiency, which contributes to muscle cramping, spasms, and reduced strength. The minerals are best absorbed and tolerated when taken with vitamin D and calcium.

Part 2: FLEXIBILITY EXERCISES

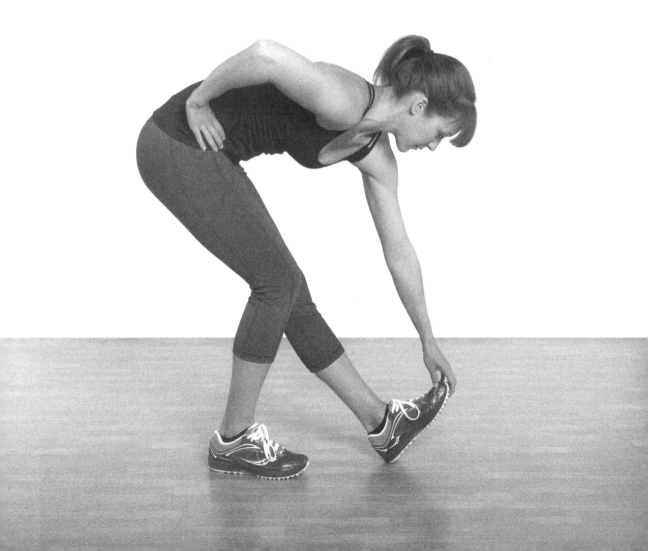

Active Stretches

Active stretches prepare your body to move through all planes of motion freely. An active stretch is one in which you move into and out of the stretch, holding it for only a few seconds at a time. One of the benefits of active stretching, also called ballistic stretching, is that it increases range of motion without decreasing power, according to a study published in the *Journal of Strength and Conditioning Research*. This is particularly beneficial if your flexibility training goals are geared toward preparing you for athletic activity.

Leg Swing

This simple exercise warms your hip flexors and helps loosen them for deeper stretching.

STARTING POSITION: Stand next to a chair or wall and place one hand on it.

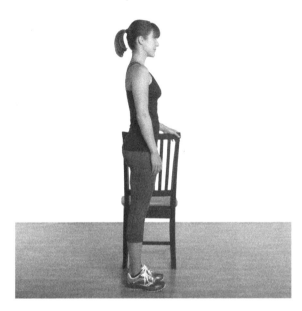

1: Contracting your abdominal muscles, lift the foot of your outer leg and swing it forward and back, keeping a neutral spine position and your hips aligned. Generate the power for the move from your hips, not your thighs.

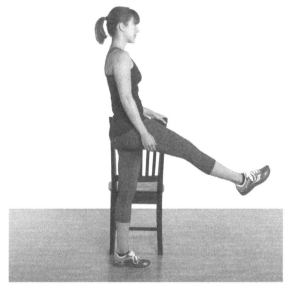

Repeat 10 times forward and backward, and then switch sides.

WHAT YOU SHOULD FEEL: A gentle warming in your hips and thighs.

Walking Psoas Stretch

It's easy to stretch your psoas muscle every time you take a step by simply extending your back leg and allowing the stretch to travel from your inner thigh into your lower back.

STARTING POSITION: Stand with your feet hip-width apart, keeping a neutral spine and your core muscles contracted.

1: Take a step forward with your right foot.

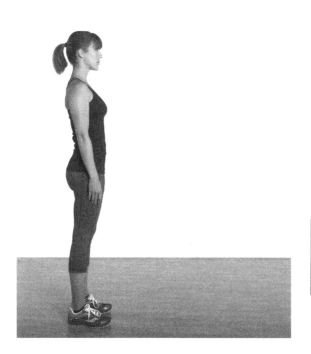

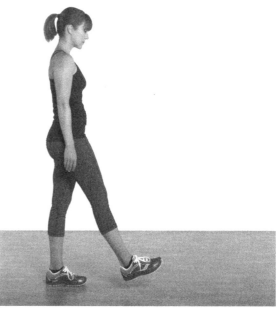

2: Leaving your left foot on the floor, extend your leg and point your toe. Keep your hips square, tuck your pelvis forward slightly, and lean your shoulders back slightly. Hold for 2 seconds.

3: Step forward with your left foot and repeat the stretch on your right leg.

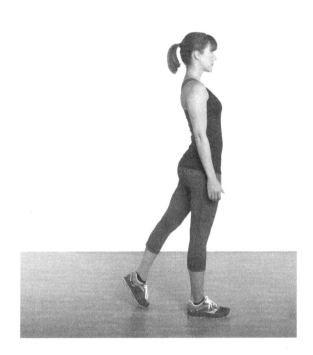

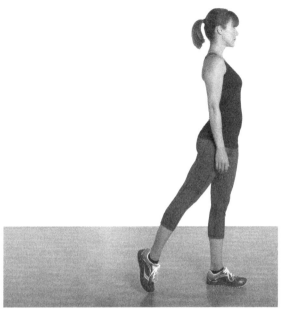

Repeat 8–10 times on each leg.

WHAT YOU SHOULD FEEL: A gentle stretch that travels up your extended leg, from your quadriceps through your psoas and into your abdominal muscles.

Kneeling Knee Crunch

One of the chief functions of the psoas muscle is to bring the knee toward the torso and chest. This active stretch improves range of motion in both the psoas muscle as well as the gluteal muscles. You may want to use a mat to protect your knees.

STARTING POSITION: Kneel with your hands directly beneath your shoulders and your knees directly beneath your hips. Your spine should be in a neutral position.

1: Keeping your hips aligned, bring one knee in toward your chest until you feel a gentle pulling sensation in your hips. Hold for 1–2 seconds.

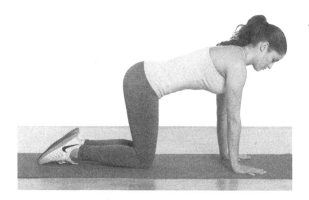

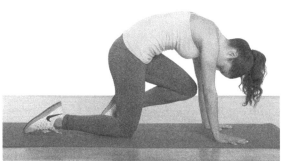

Release and repeat 10–15 times, then switch sides.

WHAT YOU SHOULD FEEL: A contraction in your core muscles and a gentle stretch in the gluteal muscles.

Lunge

This is an excellent exercise to perform as part of your warm-up and therefore shouldn't be used to push the muscles past what feels comfortable.

STARTING POSITION: Stand with your feet underneath your hips.

1: Step one foot forward, slightly farther than a typical stride length. Distribute your weight evenly between both legs. Place the toe of your rear leg on the floor and bend that knee, lowering your hips toward the floor for a count of 2. Pause at the bottom of the move. Tuck your pelvis forward, maintaining alignment in your hips. Hold for 1 count.

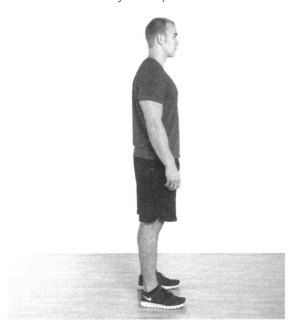

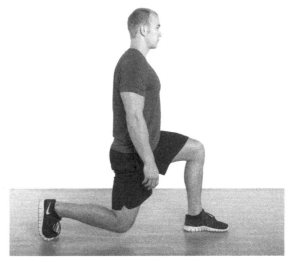

Rise to starting position for 1 count.

Repeat the move 8–10 times before switching legs.

WALKING VARIATION: Bring your rear leg off the floor and step forward, farther than a typical stride length. Continue with your other leg.

WHAT YOU SHOULD FEEL: A gentle stretch in your hip flexors, from your quadriceps into the origination point of the psoas muscle in your lower back.

Inner Thigh Stretch

Your psoas and iliacus insert in your inner thighs at the top of the femur. This stretch targets the iliopsoas from yet another angle for greater flexibility and range of motion. For a complementary stretch, perform the static Outer Thigh Stretch (page 41).

STARTING POSITION: Sit on the floor on your sit bones with the soles of your feet pressed together and your knees opened to the sides. Maintain an upright posture and keep your abdominal muscles pulled in.

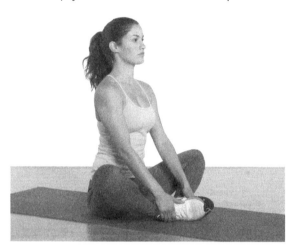

1: Place your hands on your ankles for leverage and allow your elbows to rest on your thighs just above your knees. With a flat back, gently pull yourself forward as you press your legs toward the floor. To an outside observer, you won't appear to be moving very much, but you'll feel the stretch even with very slight movement. Hold for 1–2 seconds before rising to starting position. Do not bounce.

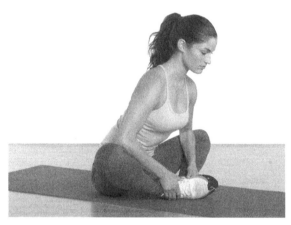

Repeat the move 8–10 times, deepening the stretch subtly with each repetition.

WHAT YOU SHOULD FEEL: A gentle stretch through your inner thighs.

Static Stretches

Static stretching involves holding a stretch for 20–30 seconds, or until the muscles release. Muscles should be warm before commencing static stretching. You can warm up with simple squats, lunges, or a brief walk or jog. The goal of static stretching is to lengthen muscles to their optimal measurement to allow them to function with ideal range of motion.

Static Kneeling Psoas Stretch

The most basic psoas muscle stretch works the psoas of the kneeling leg as you tuck your pelvis forward. It can be deepened by twisting toward the opposite leg.

STARTING POSITION: Kneel on the floor and step your right foot into a low lunge position. Both legs should be bent 90 degrees.

1: Square your hips and lift your chest as you lean forward into your front leg, extending your back leg slightly to accommodate the forward movement. Tuck your pelvis forward to feel a stretch down the front of the thigh of your kneeling leg. Be sure that your hips don't elevate or "turn out" to one side. Hold for 20–30 seconds.

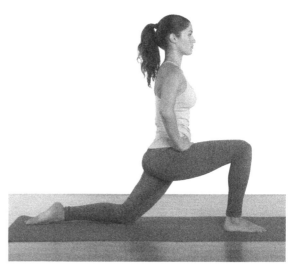

Repeat on the other side.

VARIATION: To deepen the stretch, reach the opposite arm overhead and twist slightly toward the opposite leg.

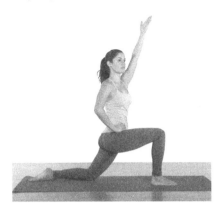

WHAT YOU SHOULD FEEL: A firm stretch in your quadriceps and psoas muscle.

Bent-Knee Stretch

When you lie on your back and elevate one leg, bringing it perpendicular to the floor or bringing your knee toward your chest, the psoas of the opposite leg will elevate your upper thigh. Allow gravity to work against this effect and increase the length in the psoas.

STARTING POSITION: Lie on your back with your legs extended and your arms resting along your sides.

1: Bring one knee toward your chest and hold it in both hands. Allow the opposite leg to remain extended along the floor, ensuring that your hips, buttocks, and thigh remain in contact with the floor.

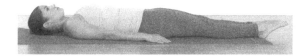

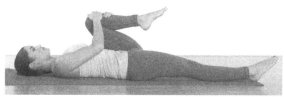

Hold for 20–30 seconds, feeling the stretch through the psoas muscle.

Repeat on the other side.

WHAT YOU SHOULD FEEL: A gentle stretch in the hamstrings of the bent leg and the psoas of the straight leg.

Hamstrings Stretch on Bench

When the Bent-Knee Stretch (page 38) no longer increases your range of motion, progress the exercise to a bench or the edge of a bed or ottoman. This will allow gravity to further pull down on the extended leg to deepen the stretch. You'll need a towel or exercise strap for this stretch.

THE POSITION: With a towel or exercise strap in hand, sit on the edge of a bench. Lie down, allowing your legs to remain hanging off the edge of the bench with your hips partially supported. Using the towel or exercise strap, extend one leg toward the ceiling. Maintain alignment in your hips.

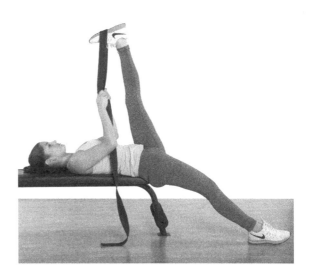

Focus on relaxing the lower leg as you hold for 20–30 seconds.

Repeat on the other side.

WHAT YOU SHOULD FEEL: A gentle stretch in the hamstrings of the bent leg and the psoas of the straight leg.

Bent-Knee Stretch on Roller

You can position the Bent-Knee Stretch on a foam roller to deepen the stretch and simultaneously release fascial adhesions in your lower back.

STARTING POSITION: Lie on the floor on your back with a foam roller placed perpendicular to your spine, directly beneath your sacrum.

1: Bring one knee in toward your chest. Grasp your leg with both hands and pull gently. Resist letting the opposite leg rise during the stretch. Hold for 20–30 seconds.

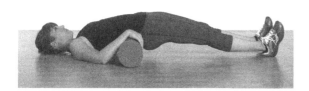

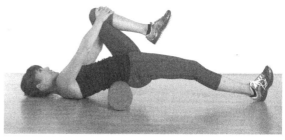

Repeat on the other side.

WHAT YOU SHOULD FEEL: A gentle stretch in the hamstrings of the bent leg and the psoas of the straight leg.

Outer Thigh Stretch

Complement the Inner Thigh Stretch (page 34) with this stretch that targets your gluteus maximus and other hip abductors.

STARTING POSITION: Sit on the floor on your sit bones with your legs extended in front of you. Maintain a neutral spine and upright posture.

1: Bring your right knee toward your chest and place the foot flat on the floor near your knee.

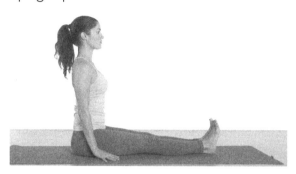

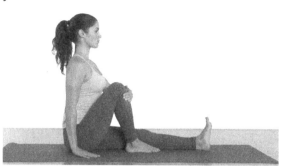

2: Rotate your trunk toward your bent knee and reach your left arm around the bent leg, using it for leverage. Support your body with your right hand on the floor behind you. Gaze slightly behind you over your right shoulder. Hold for 20–30 seconds.

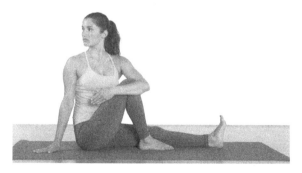

Release and repeat on the other side.

WHAT YOU SHOULD FEEL: A gentle stretch in your outer thigh.

Quadriceps Stretch

As part of your hip flexors, your quadriceps are intimately linked to the health of your psoas muscle. When they're too tight, they can increase tension in the psoas and negatively affect postural alignment.

STARTING POSITION: Stand facing a wall or the back of a chair for balance.

1: Lift your right foot behind you, bend your knee and grasp the top of your foot with your right hand. Your heel should come toward your buttocks and not toward your outer thigh. Tuck your pelvis forward slightly and keep your hips aligned. Hold for 20–30 seconds.

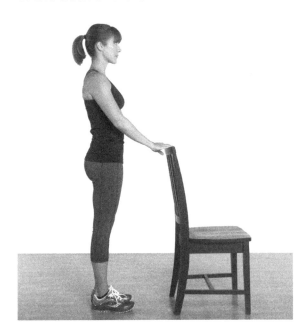

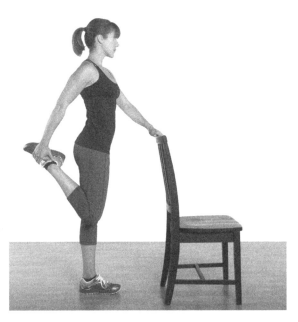

Repeat on the other side.

WHAT YOU SHOULD FEEL: An intense stretch in the quadriceps of the bent leg.

Hamstrings Stretch

Most individuals, particularly those who work in sedentary occupations or spend the vast majority of their time seated, don't need to stretch their hamstrings. Contrary to popular belief, this position puts the muscle in a constant state of extension resulting in decreased gluteal strength. It also shortens the hip flexors, which leads to an anterior (forward) pelvic tilt, further lengthening the hamstrings. However, for active individuals or those who sit with their knees in hyperflexion (feet tucked under your chair), a hamstring stretch can be beneficial.

THE POSITION: From standing, set the heel of your left foot on the floor about 12 inches in front of you. Flex your foot and point your toes toward the ceiling, keeping your leg straight. Allow your right foot to turn out slightly. Bend your back knee to lower your hips toward the floor. You should feel the stretch travel up the back of your thigh. Hold for 20–30 seconds.

Release and repeat on the other side.

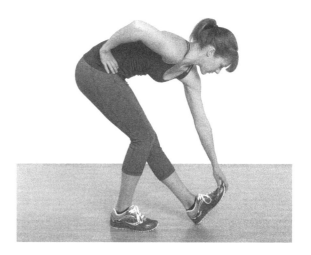

VARIATION: To deepen the stretch, grasp the toes of your front foot with the same-side hand.

WHAT YOU SHOULD FEEL: An intense stretch from the ankle to the buttocks of the straight leg.

Kneeling Psoas Stretch with Leg Rotation

Real life isn't a series of biceps curls and lunges. It's complicated, multi-joint movements in various planes of motion. Therefore, both flexibility and strength training are more effective when they recruit your muscle fibers from different angles.

STARTING POSITION: Assume a low lunge position.

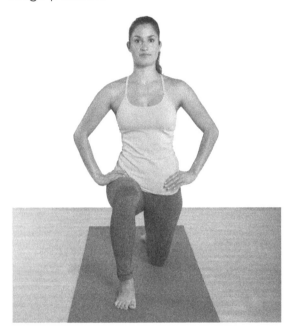

1: Bring your back foot toward the opposite side of your body so that your calf forms a diagonal line. Lean forward and tuck your pelvis forward. Hold for 20–30 seconds.

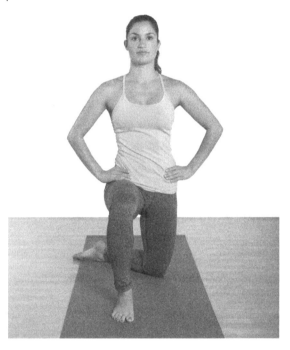

Repeat on the other side.

VARIATION: To deepen the stretch slightly, reach your arms forward, turn you palms upward, and then point your fingers toward the floor.

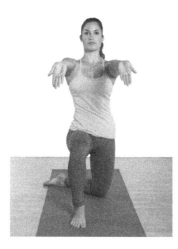

WHAT YOU SHOULD FEEL: An intense stretch from your inner thigh to your hip, closer to the groin area than a standard kneeling psoas stretch.

Kneeling Wall Stretch

When you no longer find the aforementioned stretches challenging, use a wall to increase resistance and deepen the stretch throughout your psoas, quadriceps, and other hip flexors.

THE POSITION: Assume a low lunge position with your back knee resting on a towel or cushion about 8 inches from a wall and the top of your foot elevated and pressing against the wall. Keeping your hips square, lean forward slightly. Hold for 20–30 seconds.

Repeat on the other side.

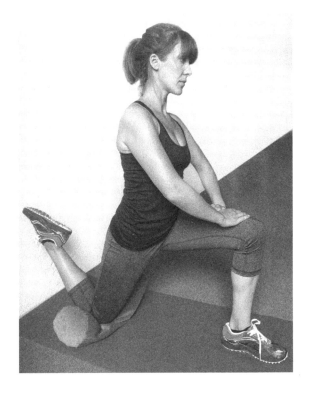

WHAT YOU SHOULD FEEL: An intense stretch through the quadriceps in your kneeling leg and a gentle stretch in the hamstrings of your front leg.

Self-Myofascial Release

Ever wish you had a massage therapist in residence? Meet the foam roller. It looks a little bit like a pool noodle but is shorter and denser. Some foam rollers have knobs or ridges on them and others are very narrow or particularly hard, but all have a united purpose: to break up fascial adhesions and alleviate muscle tension by targeting neuromuscular receptors.

Fascia isn't exactly cocktail party conversation material. However, it's important. Fascia is a thin mesh-like layer that covers your muscles and muscle fibers. Think of fascia like the fancy kitchen trash bags with a diamond-weave pattern designed to resist tears, and you have a good idea of the strength and structure of your fascia. Unfortunately, when adhesions form, they prevent your muscles from moving freely. Foam rolling breaks up these adhesions.

Fitness expert and celebrity trainer Ashley Borden incorporates foam rolling into all of her client programs. "In my almost 20 years of training, nothing has been a more crucial tool than the foam roller/PVC pipe," she says. "I've witnessed bodies of all types reach incredible results both physically and functionally when integrating rolling out into their lives."

DID YOU KNOW? *Subcutaneous fat poking up through your fascia contributes to cellulite. Foam rolling breaks up fascial adhesions, which may diminish the appearance of cellulite.*

For nearly all foam-rolling exercises, you can decrease the intensity of the exercise by decreasing the amount of weight you place on the given muscle. You can do this by supporting more of your body weight with your hands or your legs, whatever's resting on the floor.

To increase the intensity, rest all of your body weight onto a given area. If this still doesn't provide great enough stimulation, choose a foam roller that's harder, narrower, or knobbier. For the greatest intensity, use a tennis ball. This provides very targeted self-myofascial release and should be used after you have some experience with foam rolling.

While many of these self-myofascial release exercises don't target your psoas muscle specifically, they do free the surrounding muscles to support and aid the psoas in everyday movement.

Psoas Release

Tension can occur where your psoas attaches to your spine. A foam roller is uniquely suited to address this tender area and deepen traditional psoas stretches by increasing the angle between the upper thigh and torso. Be cautious about increasing the intensity of this exercise with a tennis ball until you're accustomed to "rolling out" this area.

THE POSITION: Lie on your side with a foam roller perpendicular to your body just above your hip. Bring the top knee in and place your foot on the floor, keeping the bottom leg extended along the floor. Slowly roll forward and backward very slightly.

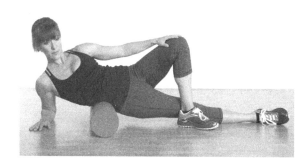

Repeat on the other side.

WHAT YOU SHOULD FEEL: The gentle stretching and moderate pain in the lower psoas of the straight leg, followed by release in the upper psoas muscle.

Piriformis & Gluteal Muscles Release

Your piriformis muscle is located deep within your buttocks beneath the gluteus maximus and is critical to hip mobility. It can be difficult to target your piriformis muscle, but a foam roller is uniquely suited to the job and can reach the entire muscle in one movement.

THE POSITION: Sit on the foam roller and place your right ankle across your left knee. Hold your elevated knee with your left hand. Lean back slightly and place your right hand on the floor. Gently lean toward your right side, placing all of your weight on your right gluteal muscle. Roll forward and back very slightly until you find the piriformis muscle. When you encounter a sensitive area, hold the position for 20–30 seconds, or until most of the sensitivity subsides.

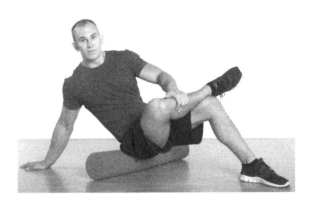

Repeat on the other side.

WHAT YOU SHOULD FEEL: Moderate pain followed by release in the piriformis muscle.

Outer Front Hip Release

The tensor fasciae latae (TFL) is a muscle of the thigh originating at the hip bone on the outer front portion of your pelvis and descending along your outer thigh.

THE POSITION: Get into a plank position over the foam roller. Roll slightly to your left side by placing your left forearm on the floor. Rest all of your weight on your left hip, just below and to the outside of your hip bone. When you encounter a sensitive area, hold the position for about 20–30 seconds, or until most of the sensitivity subsides.

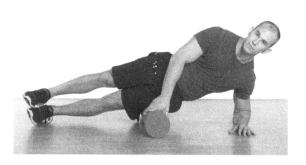

Repeat on the other side.

WHAT YOU SHOULD FEEL: Moderate pain followed by release in your tensor fasciae latae.

Hamstrings Release

Your hamstrings lie on the backs of your thighs underneath your buttocks. While most people who have jobs that require long periods of sitting don't experience tightness in their upper hamstrings, the muscles fundamental to hip mobility and health is paramount.

An added bonus of self-myofascial release technique on the hamstrings is its effect on the appearance of the skin, which can look dimpled due to fat pressing up through fascial adhesions.

THE POSITION: Sit on the floor with the foam roller underneath your thighs. Place your heels on the floor and your hands on the floor behind you. Slowly roll forward and back over the foam roller. Stop when you reach a sensitive area and hold for 20–30 seconds.

PROGRESSION: If the pressure is too light, place one ankle over the opposite knee to work one leg at a time.

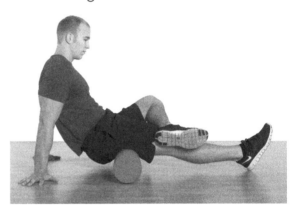

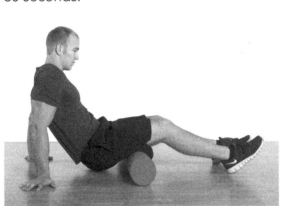

WHAT YOU SHOULD FEEL: Moderate pain followed by release in your hamstrings.

Quadriceps Release

Your quadriceps are an integral part of your hip flexors. Tight quadriceps and psoas muscles can contribute to significant lower back and hip pain as well as poor posture. This movement targets the rectus femoris, one of the four muscles that make up the quadriceps.

THE POSITION: Assume a plank position with your forearms on the floor and the foam roller underneath your thighs just above your knees. Slowly roll your thighs over the foam roller. When you reach a sensitive area, hold for 20–30 seconds until the pain subsides.

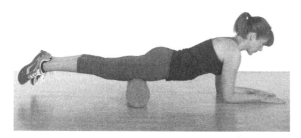

WHAT YOU SHOULD FEEL: Moderate pain followed by release in the quadriceps.

Yoga

Practicing yoga develops strength and flexibility. It's often seen as a safe, gentle form of exercise. While this is true, you should always respect your body when performing yoga. Never push yourself past the point of physical discomfort. It should feel intense, but not straining.

Achieving balance is one of the most important elements with physical activity, but especially within yoga. Thus, incorporate numerous exercises into your practice so that all of your muscles reach optimal flexibility and strength.

EXPERT INSIGHT

Yoga instructor Marlita Price shares her insight on the psoas and how yoga effectively supports psoas health.

Holistic Thinking about Psoas Health

My favorite thing about the psoas is that it literally attaches your upper body (spine T-12) to your lower body (thigh bones). However, rather than thinking of the psoas as one unit, it's best to think of it as multiple muscle groups that work together, with one set on the right and one set on left. Sometimes the strength or flexibility of these muscles can vary from one side to the other, pulling unevenly. This can lead to a sensation, as one student of mine put it, "that one leg is longer than the other."

This is why it's important to use/train these muscle sets evenly. We use our whole bodies in daily movements. Yoga is so great because the physical poses are dynamic, whole body movements that deal with the chain sequencing of action—not simply isolating one muscle at a time.

Effectiveness of Yoga

Yoga is a great way to train muscle sets evenly because there's a focus on moving in a balanced way. The mentality goes beyond making sure to do poses on both sides. By doing the poses on both sides, one can become aware of the differences experienced from one side to the other. Then, using this information, choose to spend more time strengthening one side while stretching the other or vice versa...and not necessarily spending equal time or reps on both sides.

Injury Prevention

If you have issues in the tissues, see a doctor first and give yourself plenty of time to heal before attempting an activity like yoga. Habits are formed over a lifetime so going to one class won't fix or undo them. It takes consistency and practice to first become aware of habits and then address what would be a better, healthier postural alignment for your individual needs. Avoid overdoing it to prevent what I call the "rubberband effect"—stretching too far and too quickly can cause the muscles to snap back to an even tighter, more contracted state.

Corpse Pose

If you don't consider yourself an active person, corpse pose may be the one element of yoga you naturally gravitate toward—it looks like simply lying on the floor. However, looks can be deceiving. Corpse pose, also known as savasana, involves conscious relaxation and release of tension wherever it exists throughout the body. It's one of the most important and, ironically, most difficult yoga poses. This pose is particularly helpful if you have tight psoas muscles.

THE POSITION: Lie on your back on the floor with your feet slightly wider than hip-width apart and the tops of your hands resting on the floor with your palms open and relaxed a few inches from your hips. Close your eyes and allow yourself to breathe naturally. Consciously release tension from each of your body parts. Some phrases that may aid in this process include:

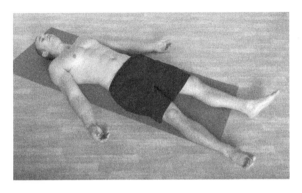

o Allow your arms to melt into the floor.

o Relax any tension in your face, jaw, and neck.

o Feel your hips sink into the mat.

o Allow your legs to stretch from your hips and feel long.

o Release stress from your fingers.

However you guide the pose, the relaxation should be allowed, not forced. Remain in corpse pose for 5 minutes. When you're ready to return to sitting or standing poses, roll gently onto one side. Slowly press yourself up into a cross-legged seated position. Allow your eyes to open gradually.

WHAT YOU SHOULD FEEL: Overall relaxation and conscious release of the psoas muscle.

Mountain Pose

After corpse pose, mountain pose probably looks like the easiest yoga exercise. But, once again, reaping the benefits from this simple standing pose requires mindful concentration. Interestingly, poor posture is one of the visible effects of a tight psoas. Use mountain pose, also called tadasana, to retrain your body to stand with proper posture. After you discover the basic pose, consider holding it while you're waiting in line or otherwise standing for extended periods of time.

THE POSITION: Stand with your feet close together, your big toes touching and your heels slightly apart. Relax your arms at your sides. Firm your thighs and consciously elevate your knee caps. Imagine a string pulling from your inner thighs, through your core, and extending from your chest and back out through the crown of your head. Press your shoulders down and back, allowing your chest to rise and your shoulder blades to relax and come closer together. Lengthen your tailbone toward the floor as you gently tilt your pelvis forward. While breathing steadily, hold for 30–60 seconds.

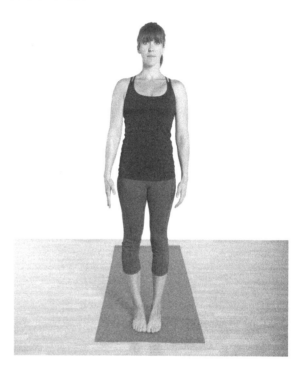

WHAT YOU SHOULD FEEL: A sense of elongation of the spine and increased strength and energy throughout the body.

Tree Pose

This balance pose develops hip flexor strength and flexibility. It also helps cultivate mindful centeredness; all of your focus will be directed toward maintaining the pose.

STARTING POSITION: Stand in mountain pose (page 57).

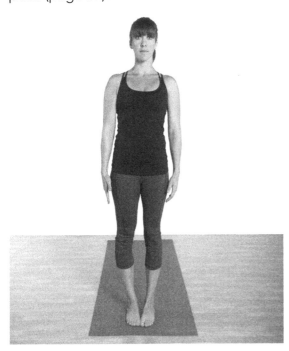

1: Lift one foot off of the floor; use your hand to grasp your ankle and guide your foot upward to place the sole of your foot on the inner thigh of the opposite leg. Your heel should be near your groin with your toes pointing downward. Contract your abdominal and gluteal muscles and tilt your pelvis forward. Breathe steadily. Bring your palms together in front of your chest in prayer position.

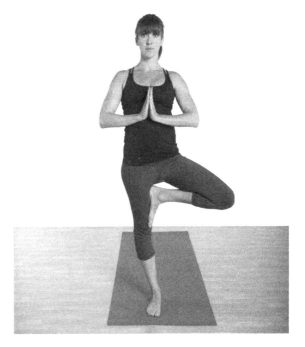

2: When you're ready, extend your arms overhead. Gaze ahead at a fixed point and hold for 30 seconds. If you fall out of the pose, simply bring yourself back into the position.

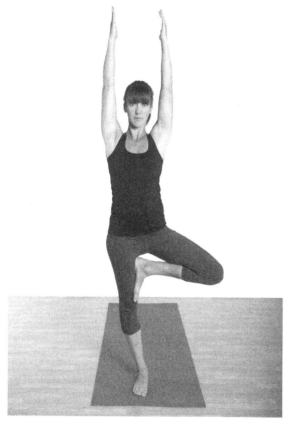

Repeat on the other side.

WHAT YOU SHOULD FEEL: An opening through your hips, a contraction in your core, and a gentle contraction in your gluteus maximus.

Pigeon Pose

Pigeon pose is referred to as a hip opener by yoga practitioners and is probably one of the most effective yoga exercises for the health of your psoas. While it doesn't literally involve "opening" the hip joint, it does loosen it to allow for full range of motion and alleviate tension. Jason Crandell of Yoga Journal *says, "Modern life requires sitting all day, which keeps your hips from the rotation, flexion, and extension they need to remain agile." He further attributes hip tension to psychological stress and common sports such as running and cycling, which can all create tightness in the hip area.*

STARTING POSITION: Get onto your hands and knees. Bring your left knee forward toward your left wrist, keeping your thigh parallel with your spine and the sides of the mat. Slowly bring your left foot toward your right hip; your shin will now be diagonal across the mat. Stretch your right leg behind you. Use your hands to push your upper body into a very slight back bend while keeping your hips perfectly level.

1: Slowly lower your body forward onto your elbows while lengthening your torso and allowing your hips to sink toward the ground. Hold for 20–30 seconds.

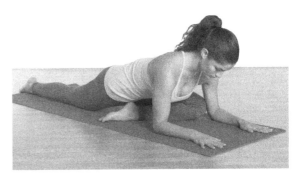

Repeat on the other side.

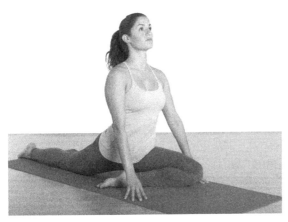

WHAT YOU SHOULD FEEL: An intense stretch in the hip flexors of your extended leg and a gentle stretch in the hamstrings of the bent leg.

Boat Pose

Boat pose requires isometric contraction of your psoas, meaning the muscle contracts to hold the position but doesn't move. If boat pose is too challenging, begin with the Chair V-Sit (page 93). This pose develops core and hip flexor strength.

THE POSITION: Sit on the floor with your legs extended in front of you. Shift your hips side to side to ensure you're resting on your sitting bones. Contract your core muscles and maintain a straight back as you lean back slightly. Bend your knees and lift your feet off of the floor as you exhale. Your upper and lower body should form a V shape. If you're able, straighten your legs and stretch your arms forward, parallel to the ground. Breathe deeply throughout the pose and hold for 20 seconds, working up to 1 full minute in the pose.

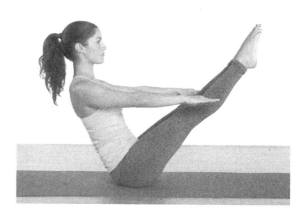

VARIATION: If this proves too challenging, allow your knees to remain bent and/or your hands to remain grounded on the floor.

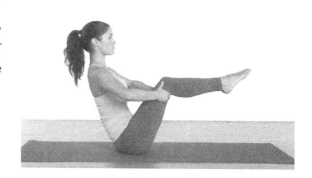

WHAT YOU SHOULD FEEL: A contraction in your lower abdominal muscles.

Bridge Pose

Not only does bridge pose require your psoas to stabilize your body, it also tones your hips, thighs, buttocks, and abdominal muscles.

THE POSITION: Lie on your back with your arms resting at your sides, your knees bent, and your feet planted firmly on the floor with space between your heels and your buttocks. Tuck your pelvis, firm your thighs and buttocks, and lift your hips from the floor until your body forms a straight line from your knees to your chest. Contract your gluteal muscles at the top of the move. Make sure to keep your neck relaxed and your shoulders resting on the floor. Hold for 20–30 seconds or longer if desired.

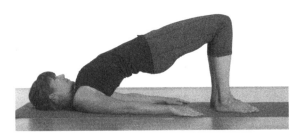

WHAT YOU SHOULD FEEL: A moderate contraction in the gluteal muscles and hamstrings.

Triangle Pose

For the psoas to function optimally, all of the muscles in the hip flexors, lumbar spine, and trunk should be optimally lengthened and strong. Triangle pose challenges your balance and core stabilization while targeting these muscles. You may find it incredibly relaxing after about 20 seconds of holding the pose.

THE POSITION: Begin in a high lunge with your front thigh parallel to the floor. Plant the back foot on the floor and turn the toe in slightly as you extend one arm forward and the other over the back leg. Straighten your bent knee while keeping the toe pointed forward. Distribute your weight evenly between your front and back legs, firming through your thighs and grounding through your feet. Shift your hips back slightly as you lean forward leading with your fingertips, as if you wanted to touch a distant object. Continue reaching until you're fully extended, then allow your body to fold sideways and your hand to reach toward the floor. If this is challenging, rest your hand on a block or on your shin. Allow the opposite arm to extend toward the ceiling. Imagine your body being pressed gently between two panes of glass; your shoulders should be in alignment, both touching the imaginary pane behind you. Gaze upward and release any tension in your torso.

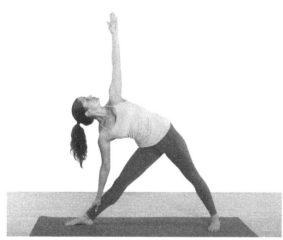

After 20–30 seconds, consider removing the block or deepening the stretch by extending your hand fully to the floor. Exhale as you rise to starting position.

Repeat the move on the opposite side.

WHAT YOU SHOULD FEEL: A gentle stretch in the inner thigh of the front leg.

Cobra Pose

Strengthen your lower back and spinal erectors with the cobra pose. While it may look like you're using your hands and arms to lift your upper body, your spinal erectors should be doing most of the work.

STARTING POSITION: Lie on your stomach with your forearms resting on the floor beneath your shoulders, your palms flat on the floor, and your fingers pointing forward.

1: Allowing your hands and arms to press gently into the floor, contract your core muscles as you elevate your chest, gazing forward. Hold the position for a count of 10 seconds.

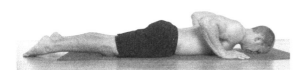 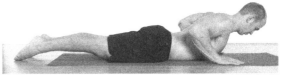

Release and repeat 1-3 more times.

WHAT YOU SHOULD FEEL: A gentle contraction in your lower back.

Crow Pose

Crow pose requires incredible upper body and core strength, balance, and focus. Your psoas muscle plays a role in bringing your legs toward your torso and stabilizing your hips throughout the pose. If you're new to yoga, consider waiting to try this pose until you develop greater strength and balance. The first time you try it, place a pillow in front of your head on the floor just in case you tip forward. Additionally, allow one toe to rest on the floor, only bringing it up once you have found your balance.

STARTING POSITION: Squat on a mat with your feet hip-width apart. Place your hands on the floor in front of you.

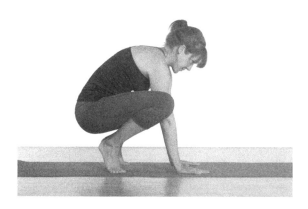

1: Bring your knees toward your armpits and rest your shins on the back of your upper arms. Round your back and gaze at the floor slightly in front of you as you lean forward. Balance on your toes until you feel comfortable lifting them off the mat to balance all of your weight on your arms. Hold the positions for 10–20 seconds, or longer if you're able. If you fall out of the position, allow yourself to rock back onto your toes and then push forward into the position when you're ready.

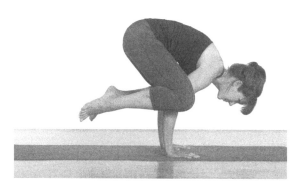

WHAT YOU SHOULD FEEL: A contraction in your upper arms and shoulders, and a gentle stretch in your gluteal muscles and hips.

Standing Big Toe Pose

This pose requires psoas strength to keep the leg elevated throughout the pose and the basic flexibility to get your leg there in the first place—not to mention balance to refrain from falling.

STARTING POSITION: Stand in mountain pose (page 57).

1: Elevate your right knee toward your chest and then reach between your legs and around the front of your ankle to firmly grasp the big toe of your right foot with your right hand.

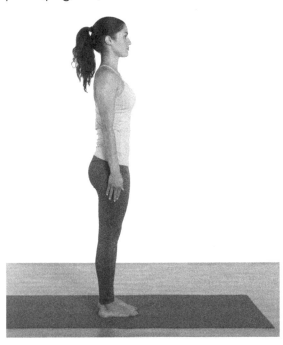

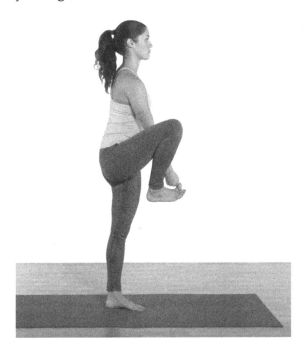

2: Straighten and lift your right leg in front of you until it's parallel with the ground. If you can, continue elevating your foot and straighten your back. Breathe steadily as you hold the position for as long as you're able.

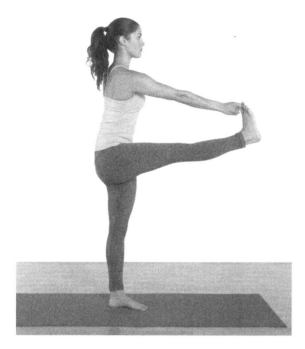

Release and repeat with the other leg.

WHAT YOU SHOULD FEEL: A stretch down the back of your leg from your hamstrings to your calf, and a gentle contraction in your quadriceps.

Pilates

In the early 20th century, Joseph Pilates created a series of exercises designed to develop physical control, strength, and flexibility. He utilized apparatuses, most notably The Reformer, as well as mat work done on the floor. In both its original form and modern interpretations, Pilates emphasizes the importance of what it calls "the powerhouse," which includes the muscles and joints from your inner upper thigh—particularly the iliopsoas—to your chest. Thus, the psoas muscle is an integral component of all Pilates work, whether or not the muscle is specifically targeted in a given exercise.

EXPERT INSIGHT: KATIE BARNES

Master Pilates instructor and celebrity trainer Katie Barnes shares her insight on the psoas and how Pilates effectively supports psoas health.

Effects of a Tight Psoas

With technology advancing further into our lives each day, normal daily movement has been greatly reduced. This is a big problem for people, regardless of their age, because of how it affects our physical functioning and postural alignment. We were made to move. It's no wonder that any new client I work with is usually suffering from the effects of a tight psoas. This may show up as anything from tense breathing or imbalanced walking patterns, lordosis, lower back pain, hip and groin pain, hamstring tightness, gluteal weakness, problems with the knee, ankle, shoulder, or neck, or any combination of these.

Clients often have specific areas of pain and tightness, like a knee, hip, or back issue, and it may appear to come from these places. However, sometimes when you follow the chain of movement that involves the problem area, you may find that a tight or overworked psoas is causing part or all of the problem at hand.

Sports and Psoas Health

As a former ballerina, I know how easy it is to overwork the psoas and hip flexors. It's usually because you start dance very young when you don't have control in your deeper core musculature, or you haven't learned how to find those deeper connections in order to stabilize and support your body. I wish I knew then what I know now! By relying on the psoas and overworking the hip flexors, you can sustain injuries, a loss of normal flexibility, and ongoing muscle pain. I've also noticed that other muscles may tend to overdevelop in order to compensate, and that sets up a constant pattern of compensation running throughout the body.

Psoas Strength or Flexibility?

I'm not a huge believer in "training" the psoas or hip flexors to be stronger, except in cases where clients have specific needs for this. Instead, I find that most people need to learn first how to relax/rest or "switch off" these muscles while learning to find and fire the deep abdominals. It helps to give people a sense or image about finding the pelvic floor and experiencing the different sensation of working obliques, rectus abdominis, or transverse abdominals. It's also helpful when clients notice that, by using their deep abdominals correctly, their midsection flattens rather than bulges out, while also lengthening the leg lines out through their hips.

I like to remind clients that they should frequently release or stretch the psoas and hip flexors after sitting for long periods and how powerful this muscle group is when functioning properly. Many see their long-term issues of pain and tightness resolved when all is well in this area.

Effectiveness of Pilates

Pilates addresses this effectively in a private session with an experienced instructor. Like with most exercise disciplines, when Pilates exercises are done incorrectly or without attention to detail, they don't help or change the client's body. In addition, many movements can lead to injury and faulty movement patterns, both of which can thwart a client's progress.

There are many reasons to do Pilates, but the main ones would be that it can change how your body feels on a daily basis and it can make you feel more open to the world around you, all while improving the other activities you do. When taking a mat class or private session, notice if the front of your hips burn for most of the class; if your knees are bent and mostly off the floor; or if you're always bending forward. These can be signs that you're overworking the hip flexor/psoas area and that Pilates routine you're doing needs a better balance of movements. Most people need more extension work than flexion exercises so it's important that, after the psoas is worked, it's released by stretching or doing an exercise that allows it to be positioned in extension.

Pelvic Curl

Learning proper technique for the Pelvic Curl is a necessary foundation for good form in further Pilates exercises and strengthens the spinal flexors, pelvic floor muscles, and hip extensors.

STARTING POSITION: Lie on your back with your arms at your sides and your knees bent, feet flat on the floor.

1–2: Contracting your abdominal muscles and buttocks, tuck your pelvis upward and draw your lower body off the floor, vertebra by vertebra, until your body forms a straight line from your knees to your shoulders.

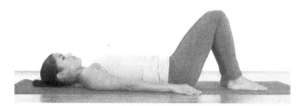

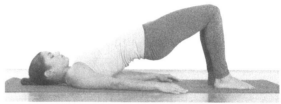

3: Gently lower your body toward the floor, allowing each vertebra to touch the floor sequentially.

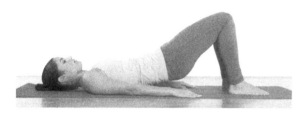

Repeat 10 times slowly and with control.

WHAT YOU SHOULD FEEL: A moderate contraction in your hamstrings, quadriceps, and gluteal muscles, and a gentle contraction in your abdominal muscles.

Supine Leg Lift

Many Pilates exercises involve lifting your legs while lying on your back. The Supine Leg Lift is a beginning exercise to develop proper lifting technique. It targets your psoas muscle and spinal stabilizers. Rael Isacowitz, author of Pilates Anatomy, *suggests imagining the cover of a heavy book being opened when performing this exercise; the cover opens without moving the remaining pages.*

STARTING POSITION: Lie on your back with your arms by your sides and your knees bent, feet flat on the floor. Throughout the move, do not allow your back to arch beyond the natural curve of your spine.

1: Retaining the knee bend, elevate one leg until your calf is parallel with the floor. Your pelvis should remain stationary, not shift side to side.

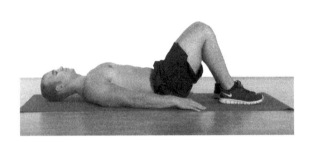

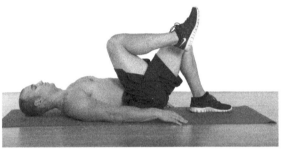

Lower and repeat 5 times, then repeat with the other leg.

WHAT YOU SHOULD FEEL: A gentle contraction in your hip flexors and abdominal muscles.

Prone Back Extension

This simple Pilates exercise strengthens the spinal extensor muscles and hip extensors, which provide balance for a strong psoas muscle. It's an especially important exercise for cyclists, runners, and those who engage in a significant number of abdominal exercises.

STARTING POSITION: Lie on your stomach with your arms extended toward your feet, pressing against your thighs.

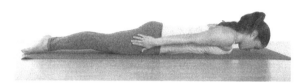

1: Pressing your legs together, exhale as you elevate your head, neck, chest, and shoulders off the floor, lifting and articulating each vertebra, arching your back and providing support with the abdominal muscles.

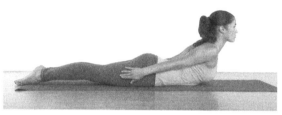

2: Inhale while lowering your upper body toward the floor.

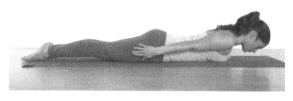

Repeat 10 times.

WHAT YOU SHOULD FEEL: A gentle contraction in your lower back and gluteal muscles.

One-Leg Circle

The One-Leg Circle targets the spinal rotators and stabilizers, including the rectus abdominis, external and internal obliques, and the transversus abdominis, in addition to the hip flexors and extensors, providing an excellent strength and flexibility exercise for the psoas and supporting muscles. The farther across the midline of your body you bring your legs, the more the hip of that leg will elevate during the move. The greater range of motion recruits your hip abductors, the gluteus medius, and minimus. Both are effective—keeping the leg inside the frame of the body will allow you to concentrate on your core muscles, whereas allowing it to extend beyond it will also engage your hips and thighs.

STARTING POSITION: Lie on your back with your arms at your sides.

1: Bring one knee in toward your chest and extend it toward the ceiling, pointing your toes. The leg should be straight, perpendicular to the floor, and directly over your hip.

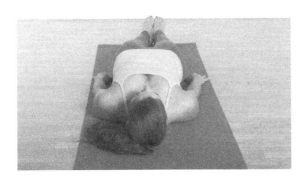

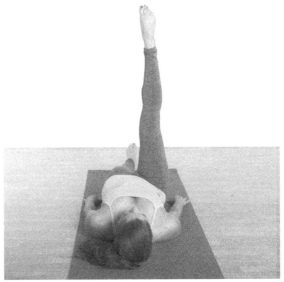

2–3: Slowly and with control, bring your leg across the midline of your body, lower it toward the opposite ankle, and then swing it back up to starting position. Imagine drawing an imaginary circle with your toe as you perform this move.

Repeat 5 times, then reverse the move by first lowering your leg, then crossing the midline of your body before bringing it up to starting position. Repeat 5 times.

Repeat on the other side.

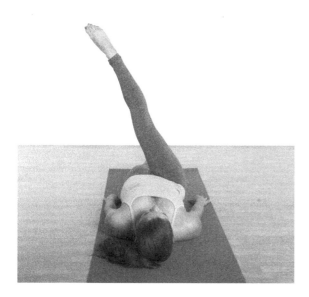

WHAT YOU SHOULD FEEL: A contraction in your lower abdominal muscles and hip flexors.

Roll-Up

Your psoas muscle and its synergists assist you in getting up from a lying or seated position on the floor. The Roll-Up strengthens your abdominal muscles while recruiting stabilizing muscles of the spine along with hip flexors and extensors to improve functional strength.

STARTING POSITION: Lie on the floor with your arms extended alongside your ears and your toes pointed.

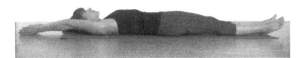

1: Contracting your abdominal muscles and drawing in your rib cage as you exhale, raise your arms and then your shoulders, articulating each of the vertebra as you come up to a seated position with your arms parallel with the floor.

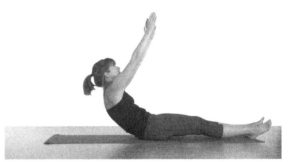

2: Continue folding forward as you flex your feet and reach toward them, touching them if possible. Hold the position momentarily, then return to the starting position.

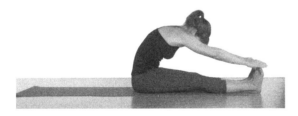

Repeat 10 times.

WHAT YOU SHOULD FEEL: A gentle contraction in your abdominal muscles.

Neck Pull

This exercise may sound a little painful but it's a very gentle move that strengthens your abdominal muscles, spine stabilizers, and hip flexors and extensors. It's slightly more challenging than the Roll-Up (page 76) because your hands are held behind your head.

STARTING POSITION: Lie on the floor with your hands underneath your head. Don't interlace your fingers; instead, stack your hands on top of one another.

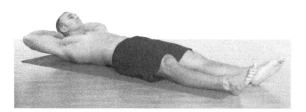

1–2: Elevate your head, neck, chest, and upper body, keeping your elbows wide. Your hands should support your head and neck, not yank on them. Continue elevating your upper body until you're seated upright.

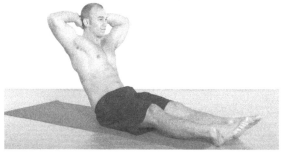

3: Exhaling and pulling your bellybutton toward your spine, fold forward, allowing your spine to round and your chin to drop toward your chest.

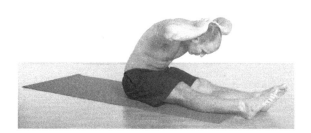

4: Rise to an upright seated position and then round your back as you lower your body to the floor, vertebra by vertebra.

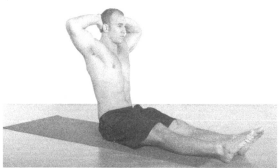

Repeat 10 times, breathing deeply throughout.

WHAT YOU SHOULD FEEL: A gentle contraction in your abdominal muscles and a slight stretch in your hamstrings as you lean forward.

Hundred

When most people think of Pilates, this is the first exercise that comes to mind, and for good reason. It engages the powerhouse and strengthens the entire body, particularly the muscles of the abdominals and hip flexors. If your head and neck feel strained, use a pillow to support them instead of allowing them to rest on the floor.

STARTING POSITION: Lie on your back with your arms at your sides. Elevate your legs until they're a 45-degree angle from the floor, turning your toes out slightly and pointing them. Draw your bellybutton toward your spine and draw your ribcage in as you elevate your head, neck, and shoulders from the floor. Elevate your arms about 4–6 inches from the floor.

1–2: While breathing steadily, pump your arms quickly in small up-and-down movements for a count of 100.

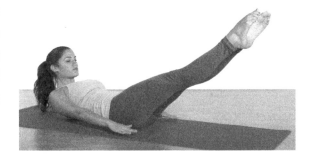

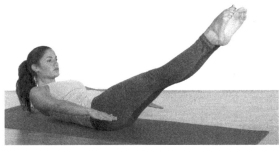

3: Bring your knees in toward your chest, hugging them with your arms. Relax your head on the floor.

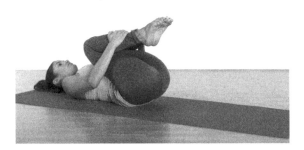

WHAT YOU SHOULD FEEL: An intense contraction in your abdominal muscles and warming sensation throughout your core.

Single Bent-Leg Stretch

Maintaining core stability throughout this exercise is challenging, requiring your hip flexors and spinal stabilizers to keep your trunk from moving while your legs bend and extend quickly. Make sure to keep your core tight throughout the move and your legs within the frame of your body.

STARTING POSITION: Lie on your back with your arms at your sides and your legs flat on the floor, toes pointed.

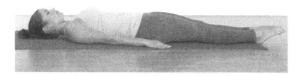

1: Draw your bellybutton toward your spine and your ribs inward as you elevate your head and shoulders. Bring one knee in toward your chest while keeping the other leg flat on the floor. Grasp the bent leg with both of your hands at the ankle and knee; give your leg a gentle pull.

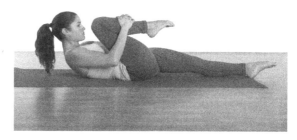

2: Simultaneously release your grasp and return the bent leg to the floor while bringing the opposite knee in toward your chest.

Breathe steadily as you complete a total of 10 knee bends and extensions.

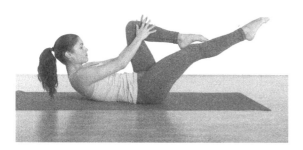

WHAT YOU SHOULD FEEL: A gentle stretch in your hip flexors and gluteal muscles and a gentle contraction in your abdominal muscles.

Single Straight-Leg Stretch

This exercise is similar to the Single Bent-Leg Stretch (page 79) but is performed with straight legs and provides even greater challenge to the core. Make sure to release any tension that forms in your neck and shoulders as you perform this move.

STARTING POSITION: Lie on your back and elevate one leg toward the ceiling. Allow the opposite leg to hover a few inches from the floor. Draw your bellybutton toward your spine and your ribs inward.

1: Elevate your head and shoulders from the floor and grasp your thigh, calf, or ankle with both hands, pulling it gently toward your chest. Make sure to keep both legs elongated and firm throughout the exercise.

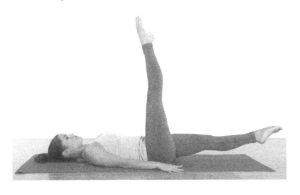

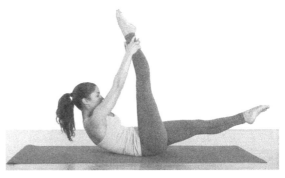

2: Switch legs, lowering the first leg almost to the floor and bringing the second leg toward your chest.

Repeat slowly 5 times and quickly 10 times.

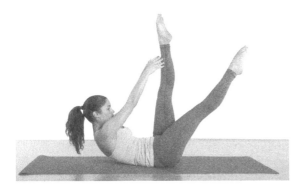

WHAT YOU SHOULD FEEL: A gentle stretch in your hip flexors and a moderate contraction in your abdominal muscles.

Double-Leg Stretch

If you want to really challenge your core and hip flexors, try the Double-Leg Stretch. At the extended phase of the movement, your psoas holds an isometric contraction to keep the legs elevated and then contracts concentrically when you return them to starting position.

STARTING POSITION: Lie on your back with your head and shoulders elevated and your knees pulled in toward your chest with your hands grasping your ankles or shins.

1: Slowly and with control, use your powerhouse to extend your legs until they're elevated over the floor at a 45-degree angle. Stretch above and behind your head, or allow them to extend toward your feet. Don't allow your back to arch during this lowered phase.

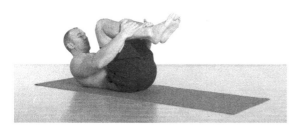

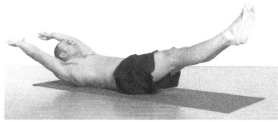

2: Use your core to draw your knees back in toward your chest, grasping your shins again with your hands.

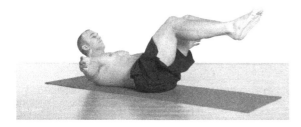

Repeat 10 times.

WHAT YOU SHOULD FEEL: An intense contraction in your abdominal muscles and a gentle contraction and stretch in your hip flexors.

Teaser

This exercise is most effective after your core muscles are strong enough to accomplish it with good form. When done properly, it strengthens the abdominal muscles and hip flexors. If you're not quite ready for the full Teaser, build strength with the yoga Boat Pose (page 61).

STARTING POSITION: Rest your lower back on the floor with your legs extended and elevated at a 60-degree angle, your core contracted, and your arms outstretched overhead toward the ceiling.

1: Elevate your torso and your arms so that your torso and legs form a V shape and your arms are parallel with your legs. Hold the position for 1 count.

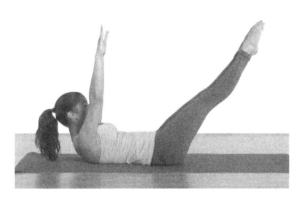

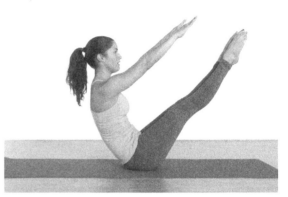

2: Lower to starting position.

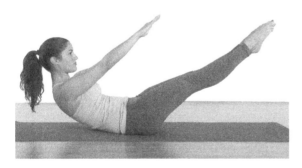

Repeat 5 times.

WHAT YOU SHOULD FEEL: An intense contraction in your abdominal muscles.

Open-Leg Rocker

Similar to the Teaser (page 82), the Open-Leg Rocker also develops balance and stability by rocking your entire body back while holding the pose. Although it might seem easier than the Teaser in that it doesn't require you to hold the starting position for long, it shouldn't be your default to avoid the challenge of holding the position.

STARTING POSITION: Begin in a V-sit position, similar to the teaser exercise, but grasping your ankles.

1: Allowing your lower back to round slightly, lean back and rock onto your back and shoulders.

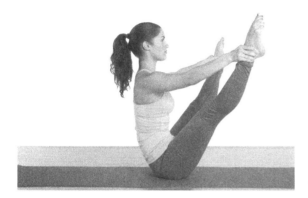 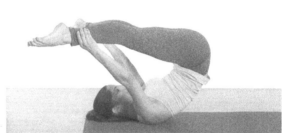

2: Roll up to starting position.

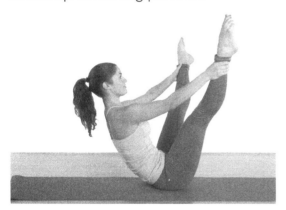

Repeat 5 times.

WHAT YOU SHOULD FEEL: A moderate contraction in your abdominal muscles and a gentle massage of the spine as you roll backward.

Rollover

The Rollover can be performed with legs parted slightly or pressed together. Either way, it targets your abdominal muscles and hip flexors, including your psoas. Be cautious performing this exercise if you have any tightness in your neck or shoulders.

STARTING POSITION: Lie on your back with your arms at your sides, your palms resting on the floor, and your legs elevated at a 60-degree angle.

1: Contract your abdominal muscles and bring your legs up until they're perpendicular to the floor.

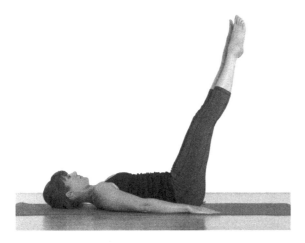

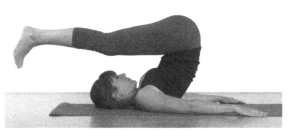

2: Round your back and continue swinging your legs toward the space behind your head. Your legs should remain completely straight through the entire move. If you're flexible enough to do so, allow your feet to touch the floor behind your head.

3: Slowly and with control, lower your pelvis toward the floor, vertebra by vertebra, until you've returned to starting position.

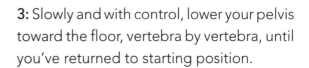

Repeat 5 times.

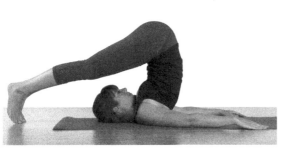

VARIATION: Begin with your legs glued together and then part them when they're touching the mat above your head. Alternately, begin with your legs slightly parted, and bring them together when they're above your head.

WHAT YOU SHOULD FEEL: A moderate contraction in your abdominals and hip flexors and a gentle stretch in your hamstrings.

Jackknife

Don't let its name intimidate you! The Jackknife is a powerful exercise for strengthening your abdominal muscles, hip flexors, and hip extensors. As with the Rollover (page 84), be cautious if you have tightness in your neck or shoulders.

STARTING POSITION: Lie on your back with your arms at your sides, your palms resting on the floor, and your legs elevated at a 45-degree angle.

1: Contract your abdominals and round your lower back as you swing your legs toward your chest and eventually upward toward the ceiling. Keep them straight and nearly perpendicular to the floor.

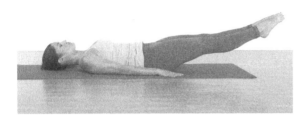

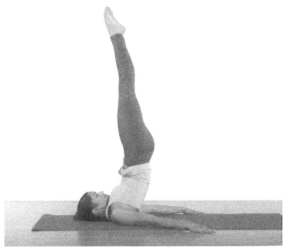

2: Slowly and with control, lower your pelvis toward the floor vertebra by vertebra.

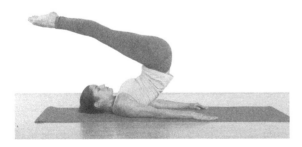

Repeat 5 times.

WHAT YOU SHOULD FEEL: A moderate contraction in your abdominal and gluteal muscles.

PSOAS Strength and Flexibility

Scissors

This exercise both stretches and strengthens the psoas muscle. It even looks a bit like an inverted psoas stretch, although both legs remain straight.

STARTING POSITION: Lie on your back with your legs extended along the floor and your arms resting at your sides. Swing your legs toward your chest, rounding your back and lifting your pelvis from the mat. Carefully place your palms underneath your hips. Your torso should form a straight line from your shoulders to your hips. Your legs should remain straight and be perpendicular to your torso, with your toes above your head.

1: Supporting your hips with your hands, lower one leg until it's in line with your torso. Switch legs.

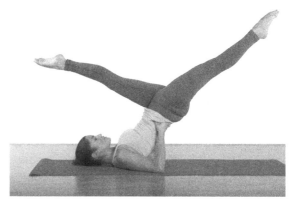

Repeat slowly for a count of 5, then quickly for a count of 10.

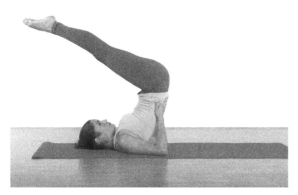

WHAT YOU SHOULD FEEL: A gentle contraction alternating between your hamstrings and quadriceps as you switch your legs.

Spine Twist

The health of your spinal rotators, obliques, and erector spinae in particular, support healthy psoas function, particularly when it comes to twisting the torso. As its name suggests, the Spine Twist encourages spinal rotator flexibility.

STARTING POSITION: Sit on the floor with your legs straight out in front of you, feet flexed. Extend your arms to your sides, parallel with the floor.

1: Exhale as you rotate your upper body, from your abdominals through your shoulders, toward your right. Hold the position momentarily, then twist just a bit farther. Inhale as you release the pose.

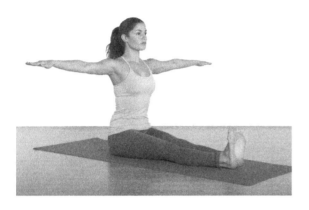

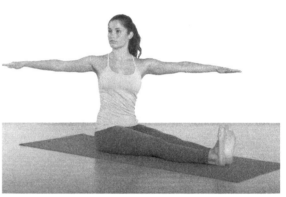

2: Exhale and twist toward your left, holding then twisting farther.

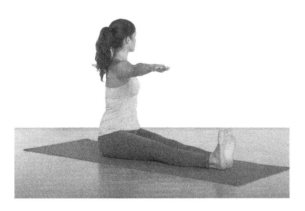

Repeat the sequence 5 times.

VARIATION: The Saw is another Pilates exercise that develops flexibility in the spine. Perform the steps listed above, but instead of keeping your upper body erect, fold forward and reach your left arm toward your right toe. Hold the position and then pulse forward to deepen the stretch. Your smallest finger should graze your smallest toe in a "sawing" motion.

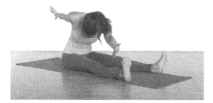

WHAT YOU SHOULD FEEL: A gentle contraction throughout your abdominal muscles.

Corkscrew

Once you've mastered the Teaser (page 82) and the Jackknife (page 86), try the Corkscrew to further engage your spinal flexors, hip flexors, and external and internal obliques.

STARTING POSITION: Lie on your back with your legs elevated over your head, as in step 3 of the Rollover (page 84).

1: Lower your hips toward one side, allowing your legs to drop toward the same side.

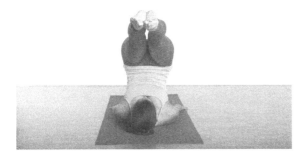

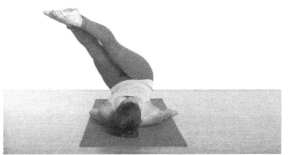

2: Shift your hips to a neutral position, circling your legs downward toward the midline of your body, then up on the opposite side until perpendicular to the floor, as if drawing a circle with your toes.

3: Reverse the move, allowing your hips to shift to the opposite side to start, then drawing your legs down, across, and up on the other side.

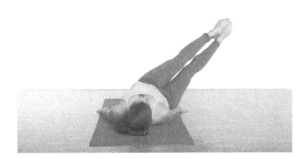

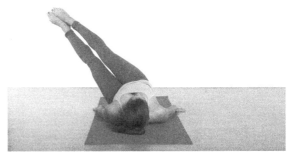

Repeat the sequence 5 times.

WHAT YOU SHOULD FEEL: A moderate contraction in your abdominal muscles.

Part 3: STRENGTH EXERCISES

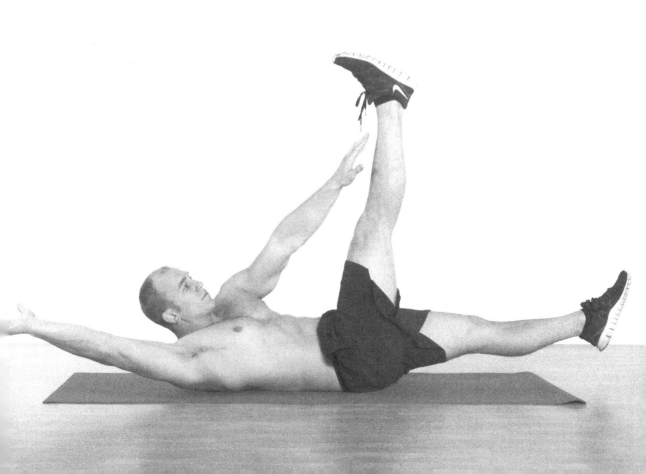

Strength Training

Resistance training can take many forms—bodyweight exercises, dumbbells, weight machines, resistance bands—and can serve many purposes. The rationale for a periodized resistance-training program for psoas health is to build strength and stability throughout your abdominal muscles, hip flexors, lower back, and gluteal muscles. This holistic approach enables optimal range of motion, prevents muscle imbalances, and reduces the risk of injury.

Periodization involves beginning with little or no load in an unstable environment to develop proprioception before gradually increasing load and altering other acute variables systematically over time. A personal trainer can help you develop a specific program to suit your needs and ensure you maintain proper form in all movements. Never jump into a strength-training program without adapting to the movement gradually, mastering proper form, and allowing your body (not a time clock or machismo) to dictate your workout.

PROPRIOCEPTION: *Self-regulation of posture and movement in response to stimuli arising within the body regarding position, motion, and equilibrium.*

Abdominal Exercises

Every time you perform abdominal exercises, your psoas gets in on the action. Whether you're doing crunches or leg lifts, your psoas' job is to bring your trunk toward your upper thighs or your thighs toward your trunk. Consequently, abdominal strength exercises require that you stretch your psoas adequately after every session. Refer to page 35 for static stretches you can perform following these abdominal exercises.

Chair V-Sit

If you're new to abdominal strength training or unfamiliar with what it feels like to contract your psoas muscle, this simple and relatively easy exercise is a good starting point. It involves isometric contraction, which means you're neither lifting nor lowering but holding a static position. You can also use a bench for this exercise.

STARTING POSITION: Sit on the edge of a chair so that your hip bones are fully supported but there's some distance between you and the back of the chair. Extend your legs fully in front of you with your feet resting on the floor.

1: Contract your abdominal muscles and lean back while keeping your back flat. You'll begin to feel your psoas contract. Hold for a count of 10.

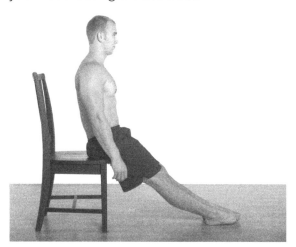

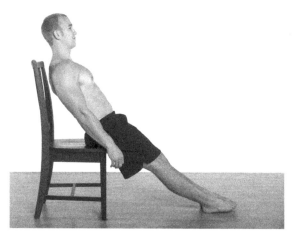

Rise to starting position.

Repeat for 3–5 sets.

WHAT YOU SHOULD FEEL: A gentle contraction in your abdominal muscles.

Scissors

Like its name suggests, this exercise involves moving your legs in a scissor-like motion. Not only does the move recruit your rectus abdominis, it also requires your psoas to contract as you bring your leg toward your chest. It differs from the Pilates Scissors exercise (page 87) in that the pelvis remains on the floor here and is elevated and propped up by the arms in the Pilates version.

STARTING POSITION: Lie on your back with your legs extended and your arms resting at your sides. Contract your abdominal muscles as you elevate both legs up toward the ceiling until they're perpendicular to the floor.

1: Making sure that your hips are square and both touching the floor, slowly lower one leg toward the floor, stopping about one inch above the floor.

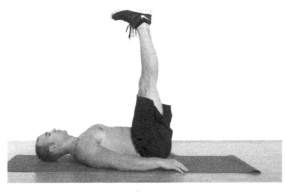

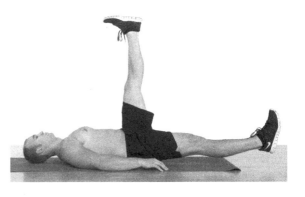

2: Raise the lowered leg.

Repeat on the other side, alternating between the two for a count of 10.

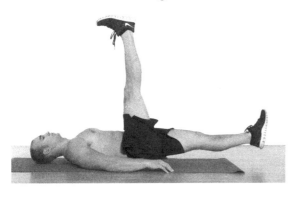

WHAT YOU SHOULD FEEL: A contraction in your abdominal muscles.

Captain's Chair

The psoas' chief responsibility is to bring the knees toward the chest, and this exercise isolates the movement, making it more challenging thanks to the effects of gravity.

STARTING POSITION: Place both forearms on the cushion rests of the captain's chair apparatus. If you don't have access to this equipment, sit on the edge of a bench. Allow your legs to hang down.

1: Contract your abdominal muscles as you bring your knees toward your chest until your thighs are parallel with the floor. Hold for 5 seconds.

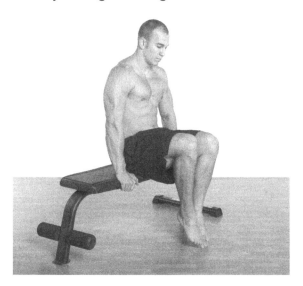

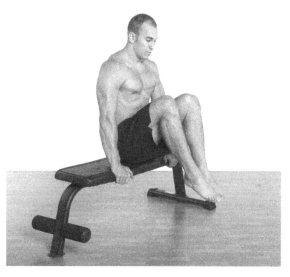

Lower and repeat for 10–15 reps.

WHAT YOU SHOULD FEEL: A contraction in your abdominal muscles and hip flexors.

> *Core stability is defined as the ability to control the position and motion of the torso to allow optimum production, transfer, and control of force and motion in integrated physical activities.*

Plank

In this isometric exercise, your psoas works to stabilize your spine. Planks are an essential abdominal exercise because they develop core stability, one of the most important reasons to train your abs. Planks are the most challenging when they're done using your forearms and elbows instead of your hands, which alter the angle to make the move easier and recruits upper-body strength to assist in the move.

THE POSITION: Lie on your stomach with your forearms resting on the floor and your hands pointed forward. Place your toes on the floor. Contract your core muscles and press up through your arms to bring your entire body into a straight position, like a plank of wood. Tighten your buttocks and don't allow your hips to sink. Hold for 1 minute, or until your form begins to be compromised or you experience any discomfort in your lower back.

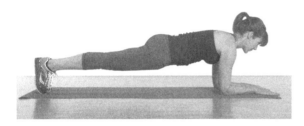

WHAT YOU SHOULD FEEL: A contraction in your abdominal muscles, lower back, and hip flexors.

Opposite Arm & Leg Raise

Your psoas is involved in bringing your trunk toward your legs and is actively involved with your abdominal muscles in accomplishing this challenging exercise.

STARTING POSITION: Lie on your back with your arms extended overhead and your legs outstretched.

Contract your core muscles, drawing your bellybutton toward your spine and allowing your rib cage to collapse slightly.

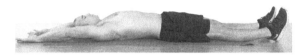

1: Raise one leg and the opposite arm, keeping both completely straight. Bring your fingertips to touch your toes or, if you can't reach, your calf.

2: Lower and repeat with the other arm and leg.

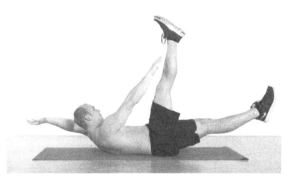

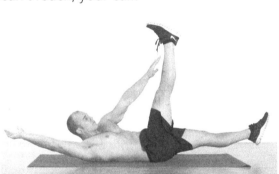

Continue slowly and with control for 10 repetitions on each side. For an added challenge, repeat the movement 10 additional times very quickly.

WHAT YOU SHOULD FEEL: A contraction in your abdominal muscles.

Russian Twist

Because the psoas muscle wraps around the hips, it's involved in the rotation of the torso. This exercise engages the psoas not only in isometric contraction but also in rotation of the spine during the twisting motion.

STARTING POSITION: Sit on the floor with your knees bent and your feet planted on the floor in front of you. Hold a moderate-weight dumbbell (10 pounds is a good starting point) slightly above your hips in front of your chest.

1: Rotate your chest to one side while keeping the weight in alignment with your shoulders.

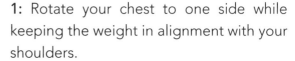

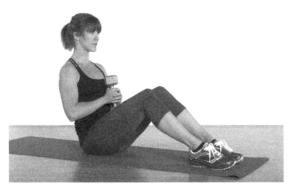

2: Twist to the opposite side, leading with your shoulders and twisting from your core for 10 reps on each side.

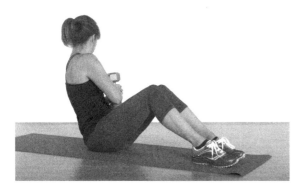

WHAT YOU SHOULD FEEL: A contraction in your abdominal muscles.

Lumbar Spine Exercises

Strengthening your lower back is an essential part of developing a balanced core, in which the psoas plays an integral role as a dynamic stabilizer.

Cat-Cow Pose

Stretch and strengthen the erector spinae with this very simple yoga move.

STARTING POSITION: Kneel with your hands directly under your shoulders and your knees directly beneath your hips. Maintain a neutral spine.

1: Exhale as you round your spine toward the ceiling, allowing your head to relax toward the floor.

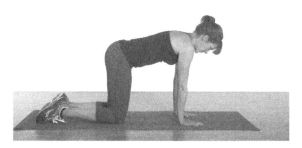

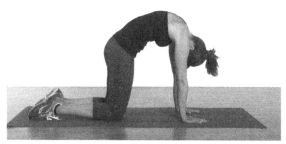

2: Inhale and lower your stomach toward the floor, arching your back gently and gazing toward the ceiling.

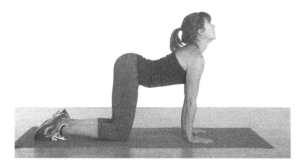

Repeat for several rounds of breathing.

WHAT YOU SHOULD FEEL: A gentle stretching and contraction throughout your abdominal muscles and lower back.

Superman

The erector spinae group, a collection of muscles that works to extend and hyperextend your back, play a critical role in maintaining proper posture. This exercise can help strengthen the erector spinae and balance strong abdominal muscles and hip flexors.

STARTING POSITION: Lie on your stomach with your arms extended along your ears.

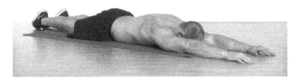

1–2: Exhale as you press your heels together and elevate your legs from your hip sockets. Hold briefly then lower your legs.

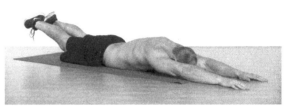

3–4: Exhale and elevate your arms, shoulders, head, neck, and chest, reaching long through your fingertips. Hold briefly then lower your upper body.

Alternate between elevating your upper and lower bodies.

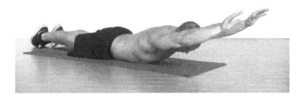

VARIATION: You can also elevate the opposite arm and leg simultaneously, or both your upper and lower bodies, for the greatest challenge.

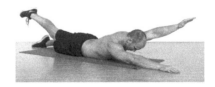

WHAT YOU SHOULD FEEL: A gentle contraction in your lower back.

Extension on Exercise Ball

This exercise is similar to the Superman (page 100) performed on the floor but requires greater strength and balance to accomplish successfully. Be sure you're very comfortable with the Superman before progressing to the exercise ball.

STARTING POSITION: Kneel on the floor with your body facing an exercise ball. Place your stomach on the ball and roll forward as you extend your legs straight behind you, balancing on your toes. The ball should touch your body between your rib cage and your upper thighs. Allow your arms to extend forward and rest on the ball or the floor.

1: Contract your gluteal muscles and core as you straighten your upper body and arms to bring them into alignment with your lower body. Hold briefly.

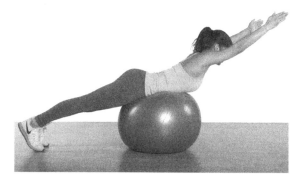

Lower your upper body toward the ball.

Repeat 10–15 times.

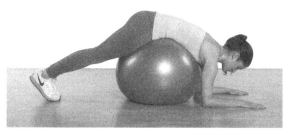

WHAT YOU SHOULD FEEL: A gentle contraction in your back and shoulders.

Side Plank

Core stabilization is a crucial element of core strength, and planks are some of the best exercises to develop it. The Side Plank in particular targets the external oblique muscles that run along your sides.

STARTING POSITION: Lie on one side with your forearm and elbow resting on the floor directly beneath your shoulder. Stack your legs and hips directly atop each other.

1: Contract your core muscles as you elevate your body into a straight line, balancing on the foot of the bottom leg. Don't allow your hips to sag. Hold for 30–60 seconds, or until your form begins to suffer or you experience any back discomfort.

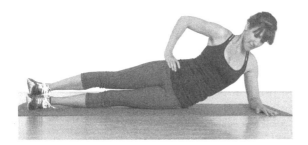

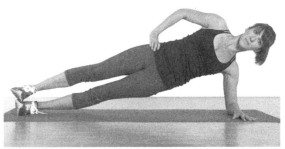

Repeat on the other side.

VARIATION: If the move is insufficiently challenging, elevate the top leg 12–18 inches from the bottom leg and extend the top arm.

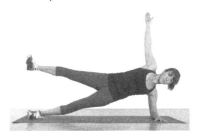

WHAT YOU SHOULD FEEL: A contraction in your oblique muscle.

Hip Exercises

Hip mobility is fundamental to the health of your psoas muscle. According to well-known primal health advocate Mark Sisson, "People have forgotten, or don't know, how to use their hips the way evolution designed them to be used. Instead of sitting back with their hips to pick something up, followed by a hip extension (thrust forward) to bring it up, they'll bend at the waist and lift with the lower back." He cites sitting as a chief culprit in lost hip mobility, which contributes to weak gluteal muscles and hip flexors, notably your psoas muscle. Regaining hip mobility and strength has the potential to reduce lower back pain and improve functional movement throughout the kinetic chain.

Dead Lift

Develop hip strength and flexibility with Dead Lifts. Initially, perform the move without weights while you learn proper technique. Although you may have done Dead Lifts before, if your form differed from what's described here, you likely weren't engaging your hips. The key is to reach your hips behind you, as if trying to find a seat, while hinging forward with your back perfectly straight. Imagine a broomstick running along the length of your spine; it should make contact with your back from your neck to your sit bones. After you've perfected proper form, add a weighted barbell to the exercise.

STARTING POSITION: Stand with your feet hip-width apart.

1: Contract your gluteal muscles, then release and reach your hips behind you as far as you can. Simultaneously, hinge forward from your hips with your back straight and reach your fingertips toward the floor. Your palms should be facing your shins, almost grazing them as you lower toward the floor.

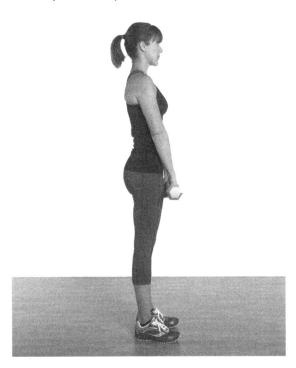

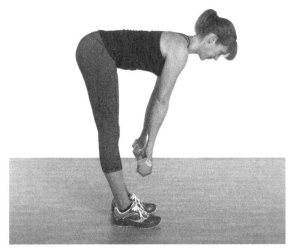

2: Soften your knees slightly and return to starting position. At the top of the move, contract your gluteal muscles and thrust your hips forward slightly.

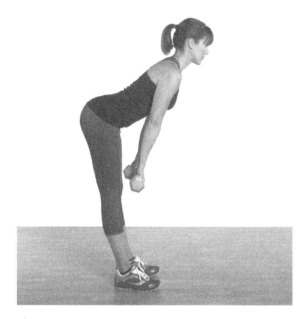

Repeat 10–15 times.

WHAT YOU SHOULD FEEL: A gentle stretch up your hamstrings and a slight contraction in your gluteus maximus.

Standing Side Kick

This exercise specifically targets your hip abductors, the muscles that draw your legs away from the midline of your body.

STARTING POSITION: Stand with your feet hip-width apart with your hands on your hips, your abdominal muscles pulled in, and your pelvis in a neutral tilt.

1: While maintaining an upright posture and keeping your hips in alignment, lift one leg to the side as high as you can.

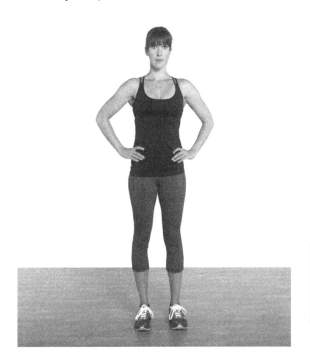

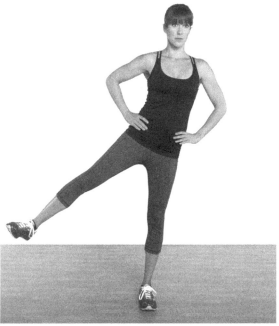

2: Lower it to starting position.

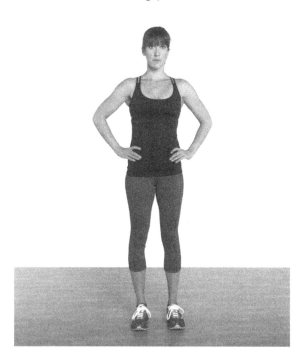

Repeat 10 times, then switch sides.

VARIATION: If this exercise is not challenging enough, use ankle weights or an exercise tube to increase the resistance.

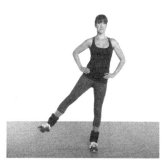

WHAT YOU SHOULD FEEL: A gentle contraction in the gluteus medius and tensor fasciae latae of the working leg as well as a slight contraction in the muscles of the standing leg. You may also feel a gentle stretch of the adductors.

Single-Leg Hip Lift

This exercise develops hip mobility while working your gluteal muscles and hamstrings.

STARTING POSITION: Lie on your back with your knees bent, feet flat on the floor, and arms resting at your sides.

1: Lift one heel off the floor and keep the knee bent as you bring it toward your chest.

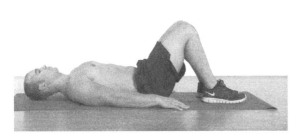
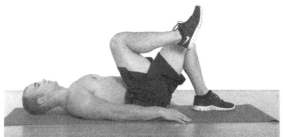

2: Elevate your hips off the floor so that your body forms a straight line from your shoulders to the knee of the leg that's still touching the floor. Contract your gluteal muscles at the top of the move and hold the position briefly.

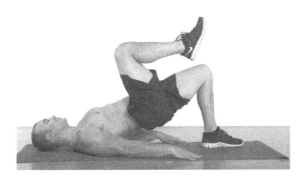

Lower your hips to the floor.

Repeat 10 times and then switch sides.

WHAT YOU SHOULD FEEL: An intense contraction in the gluteal muscles of the leg that remains on the floor.

Quadriceps Exercises

Your rectus femoris is located on the front part of the quadriceps and is part of the hip flexor musculature. It's the most prominently visible muscle in your quads, often becoming a showpiece muscle like your biceps or deltoids.

Knee Extension

If you have access to a knee extension machine at a gym, use it. Otherwise, sit on the side of a chair or bench and use ankle weights or resistance bands. This exercise develops your quadriceps.

STARTING POSITION: Sit on the edge of a bench or leg extension machine. Hold onto the sides of the seat with your hands.

1: Extend one leg outward for a count of 2. Hold for 1 count and lower for a count of 2. Repeat 10–12 times.

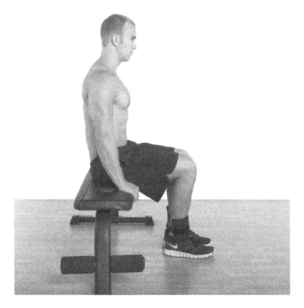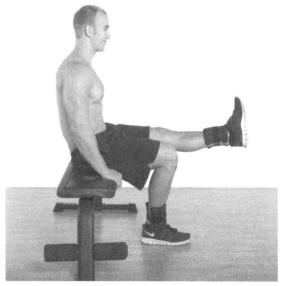

WHAT YOU SHOULD FEEL: An increasing resistance in your quadriceps.

Single-Leg Squat with Reverse Wood Chop

This exercise develops balance and coordination and challenges your quadriceps and gluteal muscles even more than the basic squat.

STARTING POSITION: Stand with your feet hip-width apart. Hold a small dumbbell (3–5 pounds) in one hand and extend it overhead. Lift the foot of the same-side leg off the floor about 6–12 inches.

1: Drop your hips toward the floor in a single-leg squat as you cross the midline of your body with the weight to gently touch the opposite knee.

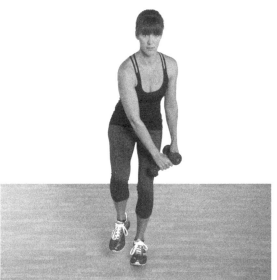

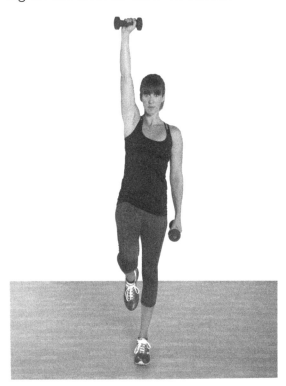

2: Stand, squeezing your gluteal muscles.

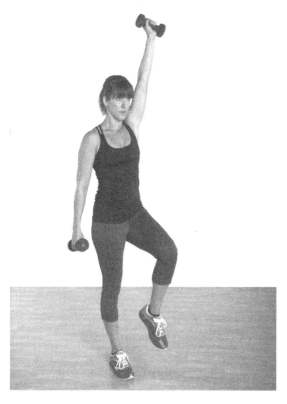

Repeat 10–12 times, and then switch sides.

WHAT YOU SHOULD FEEL: An increasing resistance in your quadriceps and gluteal muscles as well as light resistance in your shoulders and core muscles.

Static Wall Squat

Who knew that just "sitting around" could get you strong, shapely quadriceps? Try this exercise for 30 seconds, and you'll soon learn how effective it can be.

THE POSITION: Stand with your back against a wall and your feet hip-width apart. Walk your feet forward while lowering your hips toward the floor until your thighs are parallel with the floor. Contract your abdominal muscles, pulling your navel toward your spine. Hold for 30 seconds, working up to holding the position for 1 minute. Breathe steadily throughout the move.

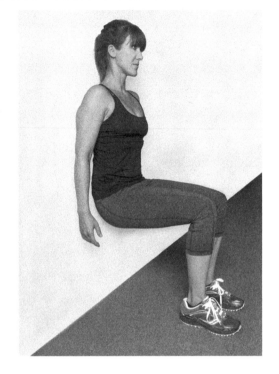

VARIATION: If this exercise becomes too easy, perform it by squatting with only one leg. Elevate the other foot off the floor as you sink down into the position and hold.

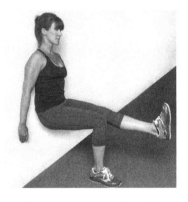

WHAT YOU SHOULD FEEL: An increasing resistance, even burning to the point of muscle fatigue and failure, in your quadriceps.

Gluteal Exercises

Sitting is particularly damaging to your gluteal muscles because it requires that they be in a constant state of extension. This contributes to muscle weakness and affects your movement pattern and muscle recruitment in other exercises, furthering the muscle imbalance. Weak gluteal muscles are often seen concurrently with a tight psoas muscle. Exercises that involve "glute activation" are an essential part of developing healthy psoas function.

So, what's glute activation? It has become a buzzword in fitness circles, but its definition remains somewhat amorphous. To put it simply, it means engaging your gluteal muscles, particularly the gluteus maximus, during exercise. In a squat or dead lift, for example, at the end of the lifting phase, squeeze your gluteal muscles tightly while holding a neutral pelvic tilt. Correcting muscle imbalances requires time and patience, but with conscious muscle recruitment, new movement patterns will eventually become second nature.

Side-Lying Clamshell

This exercise involves very little movement and its effects are equally subtle, but don't underestimate its effectiveness at awakening the gluteus maximus.

STARTING POSITION: Lie on your side with your hips stacked and your knees bent with your thighs forward, nearly perpendicular to your body. Place the soles of your feet against a wall. Your ankles should be stacked on top of one another and your toes and heels should touch the wall. Rest your head in your hand and draw your abdominals inward.

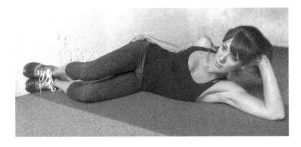

1: Lift you top knee about 6 inches from your bottom knee without allowing your hips to rock back.

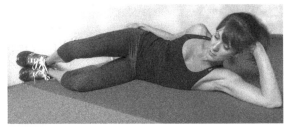

Lower your knee.

Repeat 20 small pulses. Place your hand just beneath your buttocks on your outer thigh to feel the muscle working.

Repeat on the other side.

WHAT YOU SHOULD FEEL: A light resistance in your gluteus maximus.

Quadruped Leg Lift with Bent Leg

A study conducted by the American Council on Exercise in 2006 found quadruped leg lifts significantly more effective than squats at recruiting both the gluteus maximus and gluteus medius.

STARTING POSITION: Kneel on the floor with your wrists directly beneath your shoulders and your knees beneath your hips. Maintain a neutral spine and gaze forward slightly.

1: Lift one leg behind you, keeping the knee bent, until the quadriceps are parallel to the floor or slightly higher. Imagine planting the bottom of your foot on the ceiling. Pulse the leg up, squeezing your buttocks.

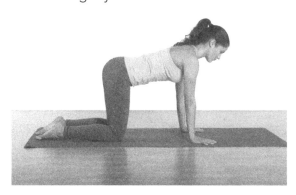

2: Lower it with control to the floor. Keep your hips in alignment throughout the move; they shouldn't elevate or turn out.

Repeat 20–30 times, or until the muscle is fatigued. Then repeat on the other side.

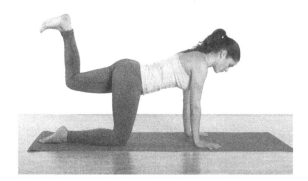

WHAT YOU SHOULD FEEL: An increasing resistance and muscle fatigue in your lower, outer gluteus maximus near your iliotibial tract.

Quadruped Leg Lift with Straight Leg

Performing the quadruped leg lift with a straight leg and elevating it slightly higher strengthens your gluteal muscles and hamstrings while providing a gentle psoas stretch.

STARTING POSITION: Kneel with your knees directly beneath your hips. Lower your forearms to the floor, keeping your elbows directly beneath your shoulders. Maintain a neutral spine and gaze forward slightly.

1: Lift one leg behind you, straightening it and pointing the toe. Keep your hips in alignment. Squeeze your buttocks at the top of the move.

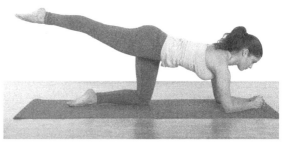

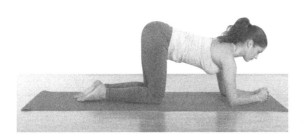

2: Maintain a straight leg as you lower your toe to the floor.

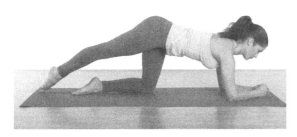

Repeat 20–30 times, and then switch sides.

WHAT YOU SHOULD FEEL: An increasing resistance and muscle fatigue in your gluteus maximus and hamstrings.

Part 4: PROGRAMS

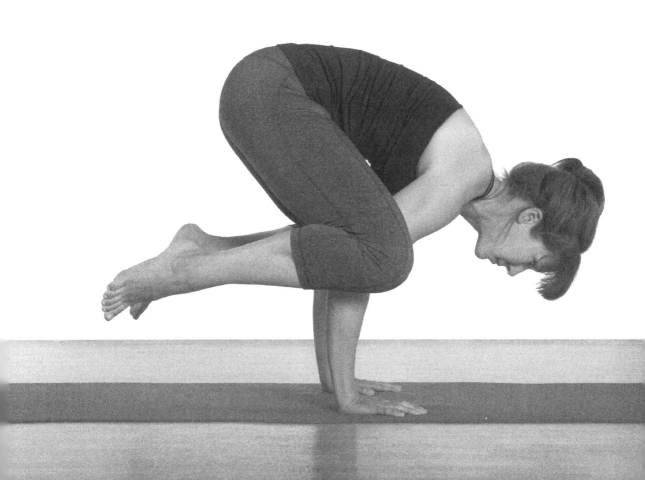

Psoas Programs

Every individual has unique movement patterns and compensations, injury history, and level of fitness ability. The following workouts provide a good starting point based on a general set of criteria. As always, never push yourself past the point of discomfort and stop immediately if you feel pain. Perform each exercise as prescribed in the exercise descriptions, progressing it as your strength and flexibility increase.

General Psoas Flexibility

You'll find a test that evaluates your psoas flexibility on page 9. If you're like most people, you likely found that it's shortened and needs stretching. This book provides a wide array of exercises designed to lengthen your psoas and surrounding hip flexor muscles, including active and static stretches, self-myofascial release, yoga, and Pilates. Start with the beginner level and then move on to intermediate and advanced as you develop greater flexibility. Perform one set of each of these exercises on alternating days of the week.

BEGINNER	INTERMEDIATE	ADVANCED
Leg Swing, page 29	Static Kneeling Psoas Stretch, page 36	Bent-Knee Stretch on Roller, page 40
Walking Psoas Stretch, page 30	Hamstrings on Bench, page 39	Kneeling Wall Stretch, page 46
Bent-Knee Stretch, page 38	Psoas Release, page 49	Kneeling Psoas Stretch with Leg Rotation, page 44
Corpse Pose, page 56	Triangle Pose, page 63	Pigeon Pose, page 60
Bridge Pose, page 62	Tree Pose, page 58	Boat Pose, page 61
Double-Leg Stretch, page 81	Extension on Exercise Ball, page 101	Scissors (Pilates), page 87
Standing Side Kick, page 106	Spine Twist, page 88	Corkscrew, page 90

General Psoas Strength

Few people need to strengthen their psoas muscle but, as stated previously, a tight psoas is not synonymous with a strong psoas. If the strength test described on page 9 reveals psoas weakness, use these exercises to increase strength. Follow them with one of the flexibility protocols listed in the General Psoas Flexibility program (page 119) to ensure you both stretch and strengthen the muscle. Perform these exercises on alternating days of the week.

- Kneeling Knee Crunch, page 32
- Crow Pose, page 65
- Standing Big Toe Pose, page 66
- Supine Leg Lift, page 72
- Hundred, page 78
- Teaser, page 82
- Captain's Chair, page 95
- Russian Twist, page 98
- Side Plank, page 102
- Static Wall Squat, page 112
- Single Straight-Leg Stretch, page 80
- Open-Leg Rocker, page 83
- Scissors (strength), page 94
- Single-Leg Squat with Reverse Wood Chop, page 110
- Side-Lying Clamshell, page 114

Psoas Strength & Flexibility for Sedentary Population

If you have a sedentary lifestyle, you likely have poor muscle definition, weak gluteal muscles, limited mobility, and a tight psoas muscle. Whether you have an office job that requires long periods of sitting, an exhaustive commute, or an otherwise sedentary lifestyle, this program will help you stretch and strengthen your psoas and awaken your gluteal muscles. Critical to achieving and maintaining psoas health is increasing your activity level. Start gradually by incorporating daily walks following a meal. Additionally, choose a recreational activity you enjoy that elevates your heart rate. Perform one set of each of these exercises on alternating days of the week.

BEGINNER	INTERMEDIATE
Walking Psoas Stretch, page 30	Standing and Walking Lunge, page 33
Kneeling Knee Crunch, page 32	Piriformis & Gluteal Muscles Release, page 50
Inner Thigh Stretch, page 34	Pigeon Pose, page 60
Outer Thigh Stretch, page 41	Supine Leg Lift, page 72
Quadriceps Stretch, page 42	Neck Pull, page 77
Hamstrings Release, page 52	Hundred, page 78
Quadriceps Release, page 53	Opposite Arm & Leg Raise, page 97
Mountain Pose, page 57	Quadruped Leg Lift with Straight Leg, page 116
Cobra Pose, page 64	Superman, page 100
Roll-Up, page 76	One-Leg Circle, page 74
Plank, page 96	Single-Leg Hip Lift, page 108
Knee Extension, page 109	Single Bent-Leg Stretch, page 79
Quadruped Leg Lift with Bent Leg, page 115	Jackknife, page 86

Psoas Healing from Pain, Swelling & Spasms

If you're enduring the effects of a lifetime of unhealthy movement patterns, this is the program for you. It will help retrain your body to function with optimal movement patterns and muscle recruitment. However, if your condition currently requires pain-relieving drugs or restricted movement, seek the attention of a medical professional before you begin to avoid exacerbating muscle imbalances or injuries. One of the most important things you can do is to stay active. This improves blood circulation, contributes to healthy body composition, and improves joint and muscle mobility. If nothing else, aim for 30 minutes of weight-bearing activity that elevates your heart rate. Perform one set of each of these exercises on alternating days of the week.

- Leg Swing, page 29

- Inner Thigh Stretch, page 34

- Bent-Knee Stretch, page 38

- Outer Front Hip Release, page 51

- Hamstrings Release, page 52

- Quadriceps Release, page 53

- Corpse Pose, page 56

- Mountain Pose, page 57

- Cat-Cow Pose, page 99

- Pelvic Curl, page 71

- Supine Leg Lift, page 72

- Prone Back Extension, page 73

- Chair V-Sit, page 93

- Plank, page 96

- Dead Lift, page 104

References

Ace Lifestyle & Weight Management Consultant Manual. *The Ultimate Resource for Fitness Professionals.* San Diego, CA: American Council on Exercise, 2009.

Addison, O., R. Marcus, P. LaStayo, A. Ryan. 2014. "Intermuscular Fat: A Review of the Consequences and Causes." *International Journal of Endocrinology*, http://www.hindawi.com/journals/ije/2014/309570.

Al-Gayyar, M. M., M. E. Shams, E. A. Barakat. March 2012. "Fish Oil Improves Lipid Metabolism and Ameliorates Inflammation in Patients with Metabolic Syndrome: Impact of Nonalcoholic Fatty Liver Disease." *Pharmaceutical Biology* 50(3) 297–303, http://www.ncbi.nlm.nih.gov/pubmed/22103753.

American Academy of Manual Medicine. "Iliopsoas Muscle Group: Psoas Minor, Psoas Major, and Iliacus." http://www.webmanmed.com/disorders/disorders_files/musclgd/lowback/14850061.html. Accessed July 30, 2014.

American Council on Exercise. "Strength Training 101." http://www.acefitness.org/acefit/fitness-fact-article/2661/strength-training-101. Accessed September 10, 2014.

American Council on Exercise. "What Is a Kinetic Chain?" http://www.acefitness.org/blog/2929/what-is-a-kinetic-chain. Accessed August 1, 2014.

Anders, Mark. "Glutes to the Max." Ace Fitness. http://www.acefitness.org/getfit/studies/GlutesStudy2006.pdf. Accessed September 8, 2014.

Ashley Borden. "Ashley Borden Training FAQ's." http://www.ashleyborden.com/training-system.html. Accessed September 10, 2014.

Bacurau, R. F., G. A. Monteiro, C. Ugrinowitsch, V. Tricoli, L. F. Cabral, M. S. Aoki. January 2009. "Acute Effect of a Ballistic and a Static Stretching Exercise Bout on Flexibility and Maximal Strength." *Journal of Strength and Conditioning Research* 23(1): 304–8, http://www.ncbi.nlm.nih.gov/pubmed/19057408.

Bandha Yoga. "Scientific Keys: Awakening the Psoas." http://www.bandhayoga.com/keys_psoas.html. Accessed September 15, 2014.

Basu, A., T. J. Lyons. June 13, 2012. "Strawberries, Blueberries, and Cranberries in the Metabolic Syndrome: Clinical Perspectives." *Journal of Agricultural Food Chemistry* 60(23): 56, http://www.ncbi.nlm.nih.gov/pubmed/22082311.

BBC. "Muscles—Skeletal, Smooth, and Cardiac." http://www.bbc.co.uk/science/humanbody/body/factfiles/skeletalsmoothandcardiac/quadriceps_animation.shtml. Accessed August 1, 2014.

Berg, Kristian. *Prescriptive Stretching: Eliminate Pain and Prevent Injury.* Champaign, Illinois: Human Kinetics, 2011.

Blomhoff, R., M. H. Carlsen, L. F. Andersen, D. R. Jacobs, Jr. November 2006. "Health Benefits of Nuts: Potential Role of Antioxidants." *British Journal of Nutrition* 96 Suppl 2: S52–60, http://www.ncbi.nlm.nih.gov/pubmed/17125534.

Breus, M., PhD. "Poor Sleep Increases Pain Risk—Especially as We Age." *Psychology Today*, http://www.psychologytoday.com/blog/sleep-newzzz/201403/poor-sleep-increases-pain-risk-especially-we-age. Accessed August 21, 2014.

Chennaoui, M., P. J. Arnal, F. Sauvet, D. Léger. June 30, 2014. "Sleep and Exercise: A Reciprocal Issue?" *Sleep Medicine Reviews*, http://www.ncbi.nlm.nih.gov/pubmed/25127157.

Cordain, L., S. B. Eaton, A. Sebastian, N. Mann, S. Lindeberg, B. Watkins, J. O'Keefe, J. Brand-Miller. February 2005. "Origins and Evolution of the Western Diet: Health Implications for the 21st Century." *The American Journal of Clinical Nutrition* 81(2): 341–54, http://ajcn.nutrition.org/content/81/2/341.full.

Crandell, Jason. August 28, 2007. "Melt Tension with Pigeon Pose." *Yoga Journal*, http://www.yogajournal.com/basics/1808.

Crone, C. November 1993. "Reciprocal Inhibition in Man." *Danish Medical Bulletin* 40(5): 571–81, http://www.ncbi.nlm.nih.gov/pubmed/8299401.

Destroy Chronic Pain. "Fascial Adhesions." http://destroychronicpain.wordpress.com/fascial-adhesions-2/. Accessed August 1, 2014.

Edelstein, J. February 2009. "Rehabilitating Psoas Tendonitis: A Case Report." *The Musculoskeletal Journal of Hospital for Special Surgery* 5(1): 78–82, http://www.ncbi.nlm.nih.gov/pmc/articles/PMC2642547.

First Physical Therapy. "Handling a Sore Psoas Muscle." http://www.firstptri.com/news/psoas_muscle.html. Accessed September 4, 2014.

FitzGordon, Jonathan. "The Psoas Major and Sit Ups." CoreWalking. http://blog.corewalking.com/the-psoas-major-and-sit-ups. Accessed August 13, 2014.

Ford, E. S. September 2002. "Does Exercise Reduce Inflammation? Physical Activity and C-Reactive Protein among U.S. Adults." *Epidemiology* 13(5): 561–8, http://www.ncbi.nlm.nih.gov/pubmed/12192226.

Furlan, A. D., F. Yazdi, A. Tsertsvadze, A. Gross, M. Van Tulder, L. Santaguida, D. Cherkin, J. Gagnier, C. Ammendolia, M. T. Ansari, T. Ostermann, T. Dryden, S. Doucette, B. Skidmore, R. Daniel, S. Tsouros, L. Weeks, J. Galipeau. October 2010. "Complementary and Alternative Therapies for Back Pain II." *Evidence Report Technology Assessment* (194): 1–764, http://www.ncbi.nlm.nih.gov/pubmed/23126534.

Gauchard, G., P. Gangloff, A. Vouriot, J. Mallie, P. Perrin. 2002. "Effects of Exercise-Induced Fatigue with and without Hydration on Static Postural Control in Adult Human Subjects." *International Journal of Neuroscience* 112(10): 1191–1206, http://informahealthcare.com/doi/abs/10.1080/00207450290026157.

Gudmestad, Julie. "How to Stretch and Strengthen the Psoas." Yoga International. https://yogainternational.com/article/view/how-to-stretch-and-strengthen-the-psoas. Accessed August 7, 2014.

Harvard Health Publications. "Blue Light Has a Dark Side." http://www.health.harvard.edu/newsletters/Harvard_Health_Letter/2012/May/blue-light-has-a-dark-side. Accessed August 21, 2014.

Henoch, Quinn. "Glute Activation." http://jtsstrength.com/articles/2014/04/09/glute-activation. Accessed September 8, 2014.

Ingraham, Paul. "Psoas, So What? Massage Therapy for the Psoas Major and Iliacus (Iliopsoas) Muscles Is Not that Big a Deal." Save Yourself—Sensible Advice for Aches, Pains, and Injuries. http://saveyourself.ca/articles/iliopsoas.php. Accessed September 3, 2014.

Isacowitz, Rael, Karen Clippinger. *Pilates Anatomy: Your Illustrated Guide to Mat Work for Core Stability and Balance.* Champaign, Illinois: Human Kinetics, 2011.

Jiang, R., D. R. Jacobs, Jr., E. Mayer-Davis, M. Szklo, D. Herrington, N. S. Jenny, R. Kronmal, R. G. Barr. February 1, 2006. "Nut and Seed Consumption and Inflammatory Markers in the Multi-ethnic Study of Atherosclerosis." *American Journal of Epidemiology* 163(3): 222–31, http://www.ncbi.nlm.nih.gov/pubmed/16357111.

Judelson, D., C. Maresh, J. Anderson, L. Armstrong, D. Casa, W. Kraemer, J. Volek. October 2, 2012. "Hydration and Muscular Performance." *Sports Medicine* 37(10): 907–21, http://link.springer.com/article/10.2165/00007256-200737100-00006.

Koban, Martin. "Psoas Stretch." Fix Knee Pain. http://www.fix-knee-pain.com/psoas-stretch. Accessed August 1, 2014.

Koch, Liz. "Learn How to Release Your Psoas." *Yoga Journal*, http://www.yogajournal.com/article/practice-section/release-your-psoas. Accessed September 15, 2014.

Koch, Liz. "The One Muscle that Does Not Need Strengthening." Core Awareness. http://www.coreawareness.com/articles/the-one-muscle-that-does-not-need-strengthening. Accessed September 13, 2014.

Lasater, J. H., PhD. *YogaBody: Anatomy, Kinesiology, and Asana.* Berkeley, CA: Rodmell Press, 2009.

Levine, J. A., L. M. Lanningham-Foster, S. K. McCrady, A. C. Krizan, L. R. Olson, P. H. Kane, M. D. Jensen, M. M. Clark. January 28, 2005. "Interindividual Variation in Posture Allocation: Possible Role in Human Obesity." *Science* 307(5709): 584–6, http://www.ncbi.nlm.nih.gov/pubmed/15681386.

Mark's Daily Apple. "How to Regain and Maintain Hip Mobility." http://www.marksdailyapple.com/how-to-regain-and-maintain-hip-mobility/#axzz3CqFVwFfn. Accessed September 8, 2014.

Mark's Daily Apple. "The Importance of Mobility: The Hips." http://www.marksdailyapple.com/the-importance-of-mobility-the-hips/#axzz3CqFVwFfn. Accessed September 8, 2014.

Mayo Clinic. "Chiropractic Adjustment." http://www.mayoclinic.org/tests-procedures/chiropractic-adjustment/basics/definition/prc-20013239. Accessed September 4, 2014.

Mayo Clinic. "Massage: Get in Touch with Its Many Benefits." http://www.mayoclinic.org/healthy-living/stress-management/in-depth/massage/art-20045743. Accessed September 4, 2014.

MedicineNet. "Definition of Proprioception." http://www.medterms.com/script/main/art.asp?articlekey=6393. Accessed September 12, 2014.

Paez, C., L. Kravitz, PhD. "Exercise vs. Diet in Weight Loss." University of New Mexico. http://www.unm.edu/~lkravitz/Article%20folder/exandwtloss.html. Accessed August 30, 2014.

Penning, L. December 2000. "Psoas Muscle and Lumbar Spine Stability: A Concept Uniting Existing Controversies. Critical Review and Hypothesis." *European Spine Journal* 9(6): 577–85, http://www.ncbi.nlm.nih.gov/pubmed/11189930.

Perry, Marc, CSCS, CPT. "Ideal Body Fat Percentage Chart: How Lean Should You Be?" Built Lean. http://www.builtlean.com/2010/08/03/ideal-body-fat-percentage-chart/#fn-1368-1. Accessed September 1, 2014.

Popkin, B., K. D'Anci, I. Rosenberg. "Water, Hydration, and Health." August 2010. *Nutrition Reviews* 68(8): 439–58, http://www.ncbi.nlm.nih.gov/pmc/articles/PMC2908954.

Ramadan, G., M. A. Al-Kahtani, W. M. El-Sayed. August 2011. "Anti-inflammatory and Anti-oxidant Properties of Curcuma Longa (Turmeric) versus Zingiber Officinale (Ginger) Rhizomes in Rat Adjuvant-Induced Arthritis." *Inflammation* 34(4): 291–301, http://www.ncbi.nlm.nih.gov/pubmed/21120596.

Regev, G. J., C. W. Kim, A. Tomiya, Y. P. Lee, H. Ghofrani, S. R. Garfin, R. L. Lieber, S. R. Ward. December 15, 2011. "Psoas Muscle Architectural Design, In Vivo Sarcomere Length Range, and Passive Tensile Properties Support Its Role as a Lumbar Spine Stabilizer." *Spine* 36(26): E1666–74, http://www.ncbi.nlm.nih.gov/pubmed/21415810.

Ros, E. July 2010. "Health Benefits of Nut Consumption." *Nutrients* 2(7): 652–82, http://www.ncbi.nlm.nih.gov/pmc/articles/PMC3257681.

Ryan, A. S., A. S. Harduarsingh-Permaul. March 3, 2014. "Effects of Weight Loss and Exercise on Trunk Muscle Composition in Older Women." *Clinical Interventions in Aging* 9: 395–402, http://www.ncbi.nlm.nih.gov/pubmed/24623974.

Stromberg, Joseph. "Five Health Benefits of Standing Desks." *Smithsonian Magazine*, http://www.smithsonianmag.com/science-nature/five-health-benefits-standing-desks-180950259/?no-ist. Accessed September 6, 2014.

Taylor, Erik. "Hip Strengthening and Mobility Exercises for Runners." Active. http://www.active.com/running/articles/hip-strengthening-and-mobility-exercises-for-runners. Accessed August 28, 2014.

Tufo, Andrea, OMS IV, Gautam J. Desai, DO, W. Joshua Cox, DO. August 1, 2012. "Psoas Syndrome: A Frequently Missed Diagnosis." *The Journal of the American Osteopathic Association*, http://www.jaoa.org/content/112/8/522.full.

University of Michigan Integrative Medicine. "Healing Foods Pyramid™—Fish and Seafood." http://www.med.umich.edu/umim/food-pyramid/fish.htm. Accessed August 13, 2014.

Vysakh, A., M. Ratheesh, T. P. Rajmohanan, C. Pramod, S. Premlal, B. Girish Kumar, P. I. Sibi. May 2014. "Polyphenolics Isolated from Virgin Coconut Oil Inhibits Adjuvant Induced Arthritis in Rats through Antioxidant and Anti-inflammatory Action." *International Immunopharmacology* 20(1): 124–30, http://www.ncbi.nlm.nih.gov/pubmed/24613207?dopt=Abstract.

Yoga Outlet. "How to Do Corpse Pose in Yoga." http://www.yogaoutlet.com/guides/how-to-do-corpse-pose-in-yoga. Accessed August 1, 2014.

Index

Abdominal exercises, 93–98
Active stretches, 28–34
Acupuncture, 18
Agonist muscles, 5
Alternative treatments, 18
Ancestral diets, 23
Antagonist muscles, 5

Ballistic stretches. *See* Active stretches
Barnes, Katie, 68–70
Bent-Knee Stretch, 38
Bent-Knee Stretch on Roller, 40
Berries: and inflammation, 20; suggested, 24
Boat Pose, 61
Body composition, 21–22
Body fat, 21–22; chart, 22
Borden, Ashley, 47
Bridge Pose, 62

Captain's Chair, 95
Cat-Cow Pose, 99
Cellulite, 47
Chair V-Sit, 93
Chiropractic care, 16–17
Cobra Pose, 64
Coconut oil, and inflammation, 21

Cooking oil, and inflammation, 20
Core stability, defined, 95
Corkscrew (exercise), 90
Corpse Pose, 56
Crandell, Jason, 60
Crow Pose, 65

Dead Lift, 104–105
Dehydration, 16
Diet, 19–25
Double-Leg Stretch, 81

Ergonomics, importance, 12–13
Exercise, importance, 13–14
Exercises, 28–116; flexibility, 28–90; strength, 14, 92–116
Extension on Exercise Ball, 101

Fascia, 47
Fish: and inflammation, 20; suggested, 25
Flexibility exercises, 28–90; active stretches, 28–34; Pilates, 71–90; self-myofascial release, 47–53; static stretches, 35–46; yoga, 54–67
Foam rollers, 47–48; exercises, 49–53
Fruits, suggested, 24

General Psoas Flexibility program, 119
General Psoas Strength program, 120
Glute activation, 113
Gluteal exercises, 113–16

Hamstrings Release, 52
Hamstrings Stretch, 43
Hamstrings Stretch on Bench, 39
Hip exercises, 103–108
Hip flexors, 4. *See also* Iliopsoas
Hundred (exercise), 78
Hydration, importance, 16

Iliopsoas, 4, 5
Iliopsoas syndrome, 8
Inflammation, chronic, 19–21
Ingraham, Paul, 17
Injury prevention, and yoga, 55
Inner Thigh Stretch, 34
Intramuscular adipose tissue (IMAT), 21–22

Jackknife (exercise), 86

Kinetic chain, 6
Knee Extension, 109
Kneeling Knee Crunch, 32
Kneeling Psoas Stretch with Leg Rotation, 44–45
Kneeling Wall Stretch, 46
Koch, Liz, 7

Leg Swing, 29
Lumbar spine exercises, 99–102
Lunge, 33

Magnesium, 25
Massage, 16–17
Meat: overcooked, and inflammation, 20; suggested, 24

Mountain Pose, 57
Muscles, 4, 5–6; illustration, 6

Neck Pull, 77
Nutrition, 19–25
Nuts, and inflammation, 20

Office work, and ergonomics, 12–13
Omega-3 fatty acids, 25
One-Leg Circle, 74–75
Open-Leg Rocker, 83
Opposite Arm & Leg Raise, 97
Outer Front Hip Release, 51
Outer Thigh Stretch, 41

Pelvic Curl, 71
Periodization, 92
Physical therapy, 17–18
Pigeon Pose, 60
Pilates, 68–90; exercises, 71–90; overview, 68–70
Pilates, Joseph, 68
Piriformis & Gluteal Muscles Release, 50
Plank, 96
Potassium, 25
Poultry, suggested, 24
"Powerhouse" concept, in Pilates, 68
Price, Marlita, 54–55
Processed foods, and inflammation, 19–20
Programs, 118–22
Prone Back Extension, 73
Proprioception, 92
Protein sources, non-meat, 25
Psoas: defined, 4; evaluating, 9–10; exercises, 28–116; function, 5–6; health, 8, 12–18; importance, 7; programs, 118–22
The Psoas Book, 7
Psoas Healing from Pain, Swelling & Spasms program, 122

Psoas major/minor, 4
Psoas Release, 49
Psoas Strength & Flexibility for Sedentary
    Population program, 121
Psoas syndrome, 10–11

Qigong, 18
Quadriceps exercises, 109–12
Quadriceps Release, 53
Quadriceps Stretch, 42
Quadruped Leg Lift with Bent Leg, 115
Quadruped Leg Lift with Straight Leg, 116

Resistance training. See Strength training
Rollover, 84–85
Roll-Up, 76
"Rubberband effect," 55
Russian Twist, 98

Savasana (Corpse Pose), 56
Scissors (Pilates), 87
Scissors (strength exercise), 94
Seafood: and inflammation, 20; suggested,
    25
Seeds, and inflammation, 20
Self-myofascial release, 47–53
Side-Lying Clamshell, 114
Side Plank, 102
Single Bent-Leg Stretch, 79
Single-Leg Hip Lift, 108
Single-Leg Squat with Reverse Wood Chop,
    110–11
Single Straight-Leg Stretch, 80
Sisson, Mark, 103
Sleep, importance, 15–16
Spices, and inflammation, 21

Spine Twist, 88–89
Standard American Diet (SAD), 23
Standing Big Toe Pose, 66–67
Standing Side Kick, 106–107
Standing wall test, 9–10
Static Kneeling Psoas Stretch, 36–37
Static stretches, 35–46
Static Wall Squat, 112
Strength training, 14, 92–116; abdominal
    exercises, 93–98; gluteal exercises, 113–16;
    hip, 103–108; lumbar spine exercises,
    99–102; quadriceps exercises, 109–12
Stretches, 28–46; active, 28–34; static, 35–46
Structural Integration, 18
Sugar, and inflammation, 19
Superman (exercise), 100
Supine Leg Lift, 72
Supplements, dietary, 25
Synergist muscles, 5

Tadasana (Mountain Pose), 57
Teaser (exercise), 82
Tests, of psoas flexibility, 9–10
Thomas test, modified, 9
Tree Pose, 58–59
Triangle Pose, 63

Vegetables: and inflammation, 20; suggested,
    24

Walking Psoas Stretch, 30–31
Water, importance, 16
Weight loss, 22–25
Wheat, and inflammation, 19

Yoga, 54–67

Acknowledgments

I am eternally grateful for the training I received from the National Academy of Sports Medicine. Its thorough approach continues to inform my perspective on movement, strength, and functional fitness.

Special thanks to Marlita Price and Katie Barnes for their contributions to the yoga and Pilates sections, respectively. Thank you to the editorial team at Ulysses, including Keith Riegert, Claire Chun, and Lily Chou, who artfully produced the entire fitness photo shoot for this book.

Thanks to my younger (but definitely not little) brother Jonathan for encouraging me to lift heavy. And, of course, thank you to my husband for always making sure I get time to exercise and write. I couldn't do it without you.

About the Author

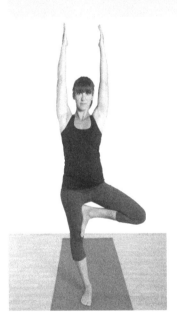

Pamela Ellgen is a certified personal trainer with the National Academy of Sports Medicine and an experienced writer on health, fitness, and nutrition. She has a passion for distilling complex scientific research into usable information for a mainstream audience. Her work has been published on LIVESTRONG.com, the *Huffington Post*, Jillian Michaels—Live Well, and the *Portland Tribune*. In 2013, she helped launch the website WorldLifestyle and served as editor of its health and fitness verticals.

When she's not writing, Pamela enjoys surfing, practicing yoga, cooking healthy meals for her family, and exploring the local farmer's market.